MIXED UP

*Combination-Feeding by
Choice or Necessity*

Lucy Ruddle, IBCLC

Praeclarus Press, LLC

www.PraeclarusPress.com

Praeclarus Press, LLC
2504 Sweetgum Lane
Amarillo, Texas 79124 USA
806-367-9950
www.PraeclarusPress.com

DISCLAIMER

The information contained in this publication is advisory only and is not intended to replace sound clinical judgment or individualized patient care. The author disclaims all warranties, whether expressed or implied, including any warranty as the quality, accuracy, safety, or suitability of this information for any particular purpose.

ISBN: 978-1-946665-48-5
©2021 Lucy Ruddle. All rights reserved.

Cover Design: Ken Tackett
Developmental Editing: Kathleen Kendall-Tackett
Copyediting: Chris Tackett
Layout & Design: Nelly Murariu

Every Drop Counts.
Every Family Supported.

CONTENTS

Why does this book need to exist? ix

CHAPTER 1

Weighing It Up 1

Liquid Gold 1
Milk Production at a Glance 2
Potential Problems with Combination-Feeding (At a Glance) 4
Why Combination-Feeding Needs More Credit 6

CHAPTER 2

The Different Types of Combination-Feeding 9

When the Mother Feels Uncomfortable or Unable to
    Breastfeed in Public 10
Where Mum Will be Separated from Her Baby and Can't or
    Doesn't Want to Express Her Milk 12
For When Mum is Exhausted and Needs a Break, So She
    Asks a Partner to Give a Bottle While She Goes to
    Sleep/Takes a Bath, etc. 16
Fear About Milk Supply During Growth Spurts 19
Because It Seems to Lead to the Baby Sleeping Longer if
    Given at Night 22
For the Non-Breastfeeding Partner to Bond 24
For Mum to Get a Reliable Chunk of Sleep Each Night 26
Mum Working Away from the Home for a Few Hours Each Day 28
Reassurance Following Early Weight Gain Concerns 30
Simple Parental Preference! 33
Baby Struggles to Gain Weight as Needed When Exclusively
    Breastfed 34
Breastfeeding is Painful 36
Mum Prefers the Flexibility of Knowing She Can Leave Her
    Baby with Someone Else 38
For Comfort Where a Baby is Mostly Formula-fed 40

During Relactation   41

Potential Problems with Combination-Feeding (and Some
    Ways to Limit Them)   42

CHAPTER 3

All About Formula   45

History   45

Formula and the Environment   49

Formula vs Breastfeeding Controversy   52

Choosing a Formula   55

Ingredients   56

Volumes   61

So, how much formula or expressed milk does your
    combi-fed baby need?   62

Preparation   63

A Word on Formula Preparation Machines   65

Storage   66

Risks   67

Dealing with Guilt or Grief   72

Human Milk and Informal Milk Sharing   77

Pros   77

History of Donor Milk   78

All About Breastmilk: How It Works   80

Causes of Low Supply   82

Human Milk Feeding   88

Volumes   90

Ingredients   90

The Benefits of Breastfeeding While Combination-Feeding   107

Antibodies   108

Oral Development   108

Comfort   109

CHAPTER 6

Combination-Feeding Due to Breastfeeding Problems 111

Why Top-Ups Are Not the End of Breastfeeding 111
Common Breastfeeding Problems Leading to Top-Ups 113

CHAPTER 7

All Things Top-Up 131

Reducing Top-Ups 131
Using Bottles 133
Hunger Cues 136
Bottle Alternatives 137
When Your Baby Won't Take a Bottle 141

CHAPTER 8

Social, Cultural, and Identity Considerations 143

Younger Parents 144
Single Parents 144
Partners 145
Working Parents 146
Pressure from Family and Friends 147
Transgender Parents and Those Who Do Not Identify as Female 148
LGBT Parents 150
Race and Combination-Feeding 152

CHAPTER 9

Making Combi-Feeding Work 159

Consistency 159
Responsive Feeding 159
Protecting Your Milk Supply 160
Tools and Troubleshooting 160
Looking After Your Breasts 164
Breast Refusal 166
Changing Your Mind 167
If You Decide to Stop Breastfeeding Altogether 167
Growth Spurts 170
Introducing Solids When Combination-Feeding 171

CHAPTER 10

**Special Circumstances: Multiples,
Preemies, Babies with Special Needs, and
Difficult Situations for Parents** 173

Premature Babies (written by Tessa Clark, RN, IBCLC) 175
Emotions 176
Twins and Triplets (written by Kathryn Stagg, IBCLC) 181
Trauma and Your Breasts/Chest 184

CHAPTER 11

Real Stories from Real Families 185

Conclusion 189

Acknowledgements 191
References 193

Why does this book need to exist?

A re you combining breast- and formula-feeding? Or considering it? If you've searched the Internet or talked to other people, you've likely found that the details are contradictory, confusing, or one-sided. Solid information is just downright hard to find.

While information for combination-feeding is out there in the world, it is often aimed at the parents who want to stop doing it. Information is also scattered widely, making it difficult to find what you need, when you need it. And you can't be too confident that it's up to date and evidence-based. This is true whether you are combi-feeding through choice, are considering it, or are mixed-feeding to help your baby gain weight while you battle milk-supply issues.

This book puts everything in one place, so you don't have to trawl the web at 3 am, wondering which article is evidence-based. It provides non-judgemental information for all parents, carers, and supporters. Whether it's to discuss wanting to combi-feed, or to talk about stopping combi-feeding in order to either exclusively breastfeed or to exclusively formula-feed, everyone is welcome here.

When I spoke to families about mixed-feeding in preparation for this book, they often told me that they felt as though they were in a sort of "no man's land" of infant feeding. They believed that breastfeeding mums looked down on them while formula-feeding mums didn't understand why someone would choose both breast and bottle. They described feeling isolated, confused, and as though they didn't fit in anywhere.

It bothers me that infant feeding is so black and white that we only ever pay much attention to breastfeeding *or* formula-feeding. So, so many families fall into a grey area in the middle, and they are mostly invisible. It is time to change that. One mum who responded to a survey I shared across my social media platforms regarding combination-feeding said:

I didn't have enough information about how to truly combination feed and so was in fear of damaging the breastfeeding relationship. I cried so much before and after introducing the bottle, thinking I was a failure, when in hindsight it was one of the best decisions for us.

I hope that by reading this book, feelings of fear and failure can be soothed, at least a little bit.

Because this text aims to offer a broad range of support, not all of it will apply to everyone. But parts of it will apply to many. Striking a careful balance between education for those who are deciding if they want to mix-feed, while also reassuring those who accept a long-term combination-feeding plan for their baby's health, is a tricky line to follow.

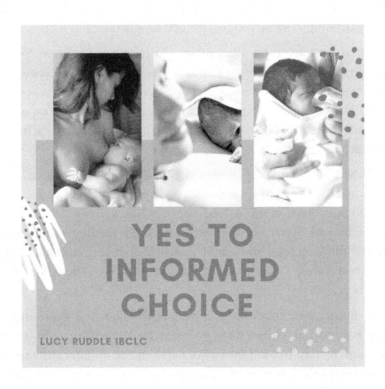

The chapters that follow are designed to be flicked through, so you can find the parts relevant to you and your situation. Combination-feeding takes so many different forms, and is used in so many different ways. For some parents, this might be the first book you pick up about infant feeding, so it seems negligent not to include gentle, evidence-based information about the power of breastmilk. Equally, I am aware that some will turn to this book when exclusive breastfeeding isn't possible, and those people absolutely must be able to access the information they need. I hope that you can take on board the parts which are helpful and relevant to *your* situation and leave out the parts that just don't resonate.

Because of the vast number of scenarios leading to combination-feeding, each section is carefully and clearly titled. If you are feeling wobbly about having to formula-feed, then you can skip the parts that might be difficult for you as they are aimed at parents who have the luxury of choice.

This book does not diminish or dismiss the great importance of breastmilk—quite the opposite, in fact. The words in these pages aim to provide information and support for families who find themselves combination-feeding, or thinking about doing so. The theory is that having access to good information all in one place may help you to provide your baby with any breastmilk for longer, and it might also hopefully allow you to meet whatever your own unique goal is with regards to breastfeeding.

Important note: The sections of this book that contain information you might want to skip are shaded, like this note! If you are struggling with difficult feelings around being forced to combination-feed, then you can skip these parts.

Jo's Story

I want to end this first section with a story from Jo. Her words are powerful and show some of the complexities we may experience regarding breastfeeding and formula-feeding. The security of keeping a baby at the breast in Jo's case was undoubtedly important for both of them. This sort of experience is why infant feeding can't always be as simple as breast or bottle. We often find mothers in the middle ground somewhere, and they need our support for a whole host of reasons.

I guess you could call me a "reluctant" combi-feeder: I had known about combination-feeding when I was pregnant, but I was adamant that I was going to be successful at breastfeeding. There's that word already – "successful." I knew from my own mother's story that she had struggled, but I was really determined to be able to feed as I knew it meant I would have to keep baby close to me and, therefore, away from my manipulative ex and his family, who lived close by. I began to find that there were lots of positives for me, and the only negative was that no one else could feed the baby – which, in fact, was a good thing for me due to my complex relationship problems.

I also thought that formula was costly and fiddly, and being that I was already responsible for everything in my household, this sounded like an additional worry.

So, the baby arrived. I didn't really know about cluster feeding or feeding responsively. I missed feeding cues in those early days and was desperate to space feeds. My ex-mother-in-law instantly suggested formula. Anyway, I did buy formula and a pump. And I started to supplement and combi-feed in the early days following his birth. I didn't use formula lots as my supply started to stabilise, but I did used to have a bottle of ready-made in my bag so that I could use it when I was out and about and felt too anxious to feed in public.

At around 4 months old, my baby's weight started to slow, and formula was given as the answer. I remember being devastated that somehow I'd failed: I then had my feelings invalidated with "oh well, you gave it a go, girl." I remember crying and my ex saying I should just give a bottle "like a normal person."

From 4 months, I supplemented with formula. This impacted my supply longer term as I was missing feeds and not expressing. I wish someone would have told me that I could do this to maintain my supply. I combi-fed until my baby was 9 months old, and my periods returned. I thought that this, plus him latching much less frequently and preferring the bottle, was a sign that I should stop. I felt fine with this.

My lifestyle was very chaotic and, as you've probably guessed, my family situation was unhappy and unsupportive: my mum was great, but she lived so far away, and she didn't share my experiences, so I didn't have anyone to really speak to. I blamed myself for not fully breastfeeding and that it was my lifestyle, chronic stress, and anxiety that had impacted my milk supply. In fact, that may have had an impact, but I now know there was more to it.

My boy fed frequently for the entire 9 months. It wasn't until many years later that it was confirmed he had an anterior tongue-tie. It also explains why it took us a while to get to grips with bottle-feeding because, of course, tongue-tie can have a huge impact on bottle-feeding too, but we did okay.

I did call the LLL helpline in the early days when I felt hideous about co-sleeping and like I'd done something wrong. This woman was incredible; she listened, supported, validated me, sent me leaflets on safe sleep and the BENEFITS of co-sleeping. I won't ever forget her kindness. I did once call the helpline after that, but unfortunately, my experience wasn't as positive, and it put me off ever calling again. I wonder, if I'd called again, whether I could have got more support with our combi-feeding?

Overall, the experience at the time was really sad and emotional, but that's because I was unsupported. The time that I had my baby at the breast was usually my safe space, time that I was needed and important, and time that I was providing for him. Unfortunately, I didn't have the best of both worlds with regards to help bottle-feeding, and still had the added life admin of making up formula and cleaning/sterilising, etc. I imagine that if my situation and circumstances were different, then being able to access additional support with feeding would have been helpful, especially given the intensity of breastfeeding a tongue-tied baby.

I look back on that time now with the understanding that he had a tongue-tie and feel sad that it was never diagnosed: it also makes me feel less "guilt" about not being able to fully breast-feed. I also think that I probably have low levels of glandular tissue, so, given the entirety of my situation, I feel bloody proud of what I'd managed to do! I feel that the act of breastfeeding really helped me and nourished my mental health and well-being in a world of chaos. Knowing that he was growing and developing how he should was really important, and with an absence of skilled support, combi-feeding was absolutely the right decision for us at that time.

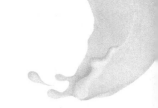

CHAPTER 1

Weighing It Up

I begin this chapter by talking a bit about breastfeeding. When I speak to parents who combination-feed, they often have as many questions about breastmilk as they do about formula. It might be that this is the first infant feeding book you have picked up, and, indeed, breastmilk is amazing! So, I'll begin here by taking you through the basics of lactation and why breastmilk is important. You might already know about this, or it might not be helpful for you right now, in which case, please do skip over this chapter if you prefer.

Liquid Gold

Colostrum is the most incredible thing. If we didn't know it was science, I would be calling it magic. What is it, and why is it called liquid gold? Colostrum is the first milk you make for your baby, and it exists regardless of what you decide about feeding. Colostrum is produced from about halfway through pregnancy as a hormonal response to the baby growing inside you. It is usually thick, sticky, and a yellowish colour, although it can be a range of colours.

Colostrum is packed with immunoglobulins, which coat your baby's digestive tract, giving the baby a shot of immune protection. Colostrum also supports their microbiome, which is set up to receive human milk. As well as this, Colostrum acts as a laxative, pushing through the thick, sticky meconium that makes up the baby's first bowel movements.

Small amounts of this amazing liquid are needed in the first few days – mere teaspoons at a time—and your body is good at making just enough.

If you are worried about producing enough milk in the early days, or you want to give your baby some supplements right away, you might want to consider hand expressing late in your pregnancy and saving any colostrum you get in syringes in your freezer. Talk to your health care provider to see if this is an option suitable for you.

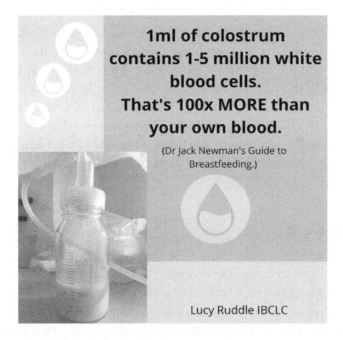

1ml of colostrum contains 1-5 million white blood cells. That's 100x MORE than your own blood.

(Dr Jack Newman's Guide to Breastfeeding.)

Lucy Ruddle IBCLC

Milk Production at a Glance

Breastmilk is made in response to emptying your breasts. The more you breastfeed or pump, the more milk you make. The less you breastfeed or pump, the less milk you make. Things that can make your supply reduce include:

- ◊ The baby having a shallow latch (this means they might not be able to remove as much milk as they need, so supply will reduce as milk is left in the breast).

- ◊ The baby not feeding often enough. We want *at least* 8 feeds per 24 hours, and a sleepy baby might not reach this goal without support to wake up often.

○ Scheduled or timed feeds. Taking your baby off the breast before they are ready may leave milk in the breast, resulting in your body slowing down production. Scheduling feeds for set times will also tell the breast to slow down milk production due to the longer than natural gaps in feed frequency.

○ A tongue-tie. This can lead to a shallow latch, among other problems, like sore nipples.

○ Formula top-ups. If we replace an at-breast feed with formula on a regular basis, the milk supply will reduce. We might want this to happen where combi-feeding is desired, but it's important to be aware of this consequence if you are being asked to top-up when you want to move back to exclusive breastfeeding.

When You're Told You *Have* to Top-up

There is nothing more frightening than watching those numbers on the digital scales flash up, having the person weighing your baby to tut or to silently write something in the health record, and then to tell you that your baby has lost weight. Again. And that now you need to top-up. It is, almost universally, a heart-sinking moment.

Further on in this book, we will take a more in-depth look at the hows and whys of topping up, but for now, I want to talk about one simple thing: does it need to be formula? Is it possible that you could express your own milk and give this to the baby? Do you perhaps need to sit down with an IBCLC or other experienced practitioner to get the baby latching well so they can remove more milk themselves? Could the baby be woken more often? Could you do something called switch feeding?

There are lots of ways we can maximise breastmilk intake before we move to formula as an alternative. Of course, if you prefer formula, then that is totally fine and a valid choice. Just don't be pushed into a decision to give it if breastmilk is your preference, and it's available.

3

A Note on Expressed Milk

I want to take a moment here to explain that this book assumes combination-feeding to mean you are using formula or donated breastmilk. If you are feeding your baby your own milk in a bottle or a cup or any other way, then you are exclusively breastfeeding. However, many parts of this book will still be relevant, so do read on. It's probably helpful for you to know that topping up with your own pumped milk isn't the same as combination-feeding.

Potential Problems with Combination-Feeding (At a Glance)

I believe that combination-feeding can work well; that's why I've written this book. However, there are potential problems, and it's important to mention them. This section gives a brief overview only, as these issues are discussed in more depth throughout the book.

◊ Milk supply might reduce more than you want it to.

◊ You may develop blocked ducts, mastitis, or an abscess.

◊ The baby may find it hard to switch between breast and bottle.

◊ The baby may refuse to take a bottle.

◊ The baby might have an allergic reaction to formula.

◊ The baby may be more gassy or windy when given bottles.

Lori-Anne's Story

I'd like to end this chapter with Lori-Anne's story because it demonstrates how combination-feeding is sometimes a choice made due to the lack of more support and information.

My name is Lori-Anne from Australia. I'm a mother of three children and a stepmother of two. My combination-feeding story comes to you from my first time becoming a mother.

I was 23 years old when I had my first child. I always knew I wanted to breastfeed my children. However, I really struggled. I didn't have a lot of help. My partner at the time (the child's father) was all for being able to feed a bottle to our child so "he could be involved."

I was young, didn't have strong support from local nurses/midwives after I left hospital, and I certainly wasn't directed to the Australian Breastfeeding Association (who, by the way, I think are amazing).

I struggled through breastfeeding for four months before I started combination-feeding. My child was feeding every three hours, and took an hour to an hour and a half to feed. I was exhausted. So began the combination-feeding. So began the slippery slope of decline in supply (unbeknown to me), and an increase to formula feeds (no one had told me about expressing, although who knows how I would have gone, I could express hardly anything with my two youngest children).

By 6 months of age, my child was fully formula-fed and had started on solids.

Looking back now, it is my firm belief that my child had (has) a tongue-tie (my now-4-year-old had ties, they were revised and I fed her until 2.5 years, also combo fed her until the ties were revised at 10 weeks old) and with limited support, combination-feeding lead to fully formula-fed.

It seems important to explore what exactly leads parents to feed both breastmilk and formula to their baby. It seems fairly clear that mixed feeding often happens because there is an understanding regarding the importance of breastmilk and breastfeeding. Still, for whatever reason, full breastfeeding is either not possible or not desired. There are many reasons for this, ranging from a lack of good support for breastfeeding challenges, physiological issues for Mum, lifestyle circumstances, or simple preference. Regardless of the reason, combination-feeding should be supported with the same good information and non-judgement that I expect and aim to offer for breastfeeding or formula-feeding.

Why Combination-Feeding Needs More Credit

There are a couple of reasons why I think that combi-feeding deserves its own space in the infant feeding world.

1. Any breastmilk feeding is beneficial to the baby and mum. The website *Kellymom* cites 50 ml of breastmilk a day as enough to have a positive impact. The Iowa Extension Service tells us that a single teaspoon of breastmilk contains over three million germ-killing cells. When combination-feeding becomes an option instead of simply "breastfeed or formula-feed," we potentially give many, many more babies access to human milk than before.

2. When breastfeeding is difficult or overwhelming, bringing in some bottles of formula or donor milk can help many a family to work through their challenges. I can't tell you how many times the parents I work with decide to give a bottle or two over a few days while nipples heal or everyone just gets their head in the game, and a month later, the baby is exclusively at the breast again. I have even supported mums who only wanted to feed their baby colostrum, using lots of bottles in the earliest days, and they have ended up breastfeeding well into the child's toddler years.

Comments from my mixed feeding survey about what families found positive included:

> It enabled me to continue to breastfeed.

> My husband was a police officer and was either away a lot or on shifts. It gave him a chance to bond with the baby when he came home, and after severe PND, mastitis, and being exhausted on my own, it gave my body a break once a day.

> It saved my sanity. Not that I ever wanted to escape, but it made me feel that I wasn't tied to home, and I could go out if needed - only to the shops or something, never anywhere glamorous!

What I found especially interesting about this survey is that a lot of studies tell us that combination-feeding leads to shorter breast-feeding duration overall. But over 40% of my respondents told me that combination-feeding meant their baby was breastfed for longer than they would have been if exclusive breastfeeding was the only option given. Only 20% said they weren't sure which way things would have gone if combi-feeding was not an option.

Combination-feeding could be an occasional bottle a few times a week or less, or it could be daily top-ups of formula equating to much of the baby's intake. The type of combination-feeding tells us more about why it might be happening.

In subsequent chapters, I explore some of these situations. However, an obvious reason for combination-feeding in any form is simply choice. We often forget this when discussing the reasons for topping up. But it is just as important as any of the other reasons I describe.

CHAPTER 2

The Different Types of Combination-Feeding

Y̶ou will notice that the sections in this chapter are divided into subcategories.

Quick glance alternatives to consider: You may not be aware of the options available to you, so this section covers those briefly. The subheading does not exist to tell you what to do; it's simply there, so you know what all your choices are.

Why you might want to give a bottle: This is a more in-depth look at why people choose to combi-feed under each scenario. Where possible, I will share studies and experiences from families here. Please also note that I use the term bottle feeding as this is the most common scenario, but you might consider using a cup, spoon or finger feeding instead.

Make it work for you: This is a boxed section that tells you how to combi-feed for your particular situation. Again, it is a simple summary, but you will find more depth throughout the book, and I will direct you to the correct page for more detailed reading if you need it.

Things to be aware of: This subcategory gives you a rundown of the potential problems you might come across. I have included this in the name of informed choice. If you know the pitfalls, you can be alert to them. I have coded these sections in pink so you can see them easily and avoid if you feel that would be better for your situation.

Occasional bottles: Giving bottles a few times a week or less often were the least common options in a survey where I asked parents about combination-feeding. Only 7% indicated that they mixed fed by offering bottles less than once a week, and a little more than 8% said they gave bottles "once or twice a week," but it still deserves to be discussed. Below, I talk about some of the reasons for occasional, *ad hoc* mixed feeds.

When the Mother Feels Uncomfortable or Unable to Breastfeed in Public

Quick Glance Alternatives to Consider

- Practise breastfeeding in public with a friend who is also breastfeeding.

- Have an idea of where in your area is considered breastfeeding friendly, and plan to go there if the baby needs to feed.

- Some mums might choose to breastfeed in their car.

- Choose a quiet corner near the back of a coffee shop if you are anxious.

I felt much more confident knowing I could give her a bottle if she was fussy when we were out in public.

~ Carly

Why You Might Want to Combi-Feed

Anxiety or fear about breastfeeding in public is common in the West. A study in 2005 by Hannan et al. asked Americans across different states if they felt mothers should have a right to breastfeed in public.

> …agreement with the statement "I believe women should have the right to breastfeed in public" ranged from 37.2% in the East South-Central region to 58.8% in the Mountain region.

The *UK Infant Feeding Survey 2010* found that 40% of mothers had never breastfed in public.

So, it's hardly surprising that mothers may decide to use bottles while they are out and about in public. Having said this, 80% of women using a breastfeeding in public review app reported positive experiences when nursing in public (Simpson et al., 2016).

A *SummerStyles* Survey carried out in the US in 2018 found only 10.5% of participants disagreed with the statement, "I believe women should have the right to breastfeed in public spaces." So, some data suggests that the tides are turning with regard to public opinion.

MAKING IT WORK

◊   Make sure you have everything you need ready to go. A flask of hot water, your milk powder, and a clean bottle. Or your expressed milk in a cool bag, and a flask of hot water to warm it if your baby won't take milk cold.

◊   If you are only going to be missing one breastfeed, and this isn't happening several days a week, then supply is unlikely to be a worry, but you may need to express or feed as soon as you get home or back to your car if your breasts are very full.

◊   Paced bottle-feeding may help avoid overfeeding and bottle preference.

Some Things to be Aware of if You Want to Give a Bottle When Out in Public

The baby may simply sleep while you are out!

You may find that your breasts become full, and you can't relieve them easily if you are not at home.

The baby may not take the bottle if one is not given often.

You might find that the baby goes longer than expected between a bottle-feed and breastfeed, making those full breasts potentially even more problematic.

The baby may still want to breastfeed after a bottle, as they might want the comfort and reassurance of your breast.

Breastfeeding in the UK and the U. S. is protected by law. This means you have every right to breastfeed in public as long as you are not causing a risk or obstruction. No one can make you stop or move.

Where Mum Will be Separated from Her Baby and Can't or Doesn't Want to Express Her Milk

Quick Glance Alternatives to Consider

- ◊ Can the baby go with Mum, even if this would mean a carer looks after the baby in between feeds?

"I left him for six hours to go to a close friend's wedding. Knowing how to hand express was a life saver!! It was fantastic to be able to let my hair down for a day and be "me" again without worrying about my baby. I was glad to get back to him though!"

~ Jazz

Why You Might Want to Combi-Feed

Some women struggle to express either by hand or with a pump. No matter how hard they try, they say that little seems to happen. However, start to dig a little deeper, and often it turns out that the mother is expressing a normal and expected amount of milk. If the parent doesn't know this, though, they can become disheartened or worried that the baby won't be getting enough milk when separated for several hours. A bottle of formula can seem like the easiest solution to this problem.

It is normal to only see 20 ml or 30 ml in the bottle when expressing, but over several days of expressing, this will build to a couple of feeds ready to give to the baby. Furthermore, milk that has been expressed on one day can be added to milk expressed a day or two ago once both containers reach the same fridge temperature.

Average volumes per hour of separation are also surprisingly small, with sources suggesting between 1-1.5 oz.

However, some mothers who attach a breast pump find that genuinely nothing happens. A breast pump is nothing like a baby, really. Even the way in which it removes milk is different from how a baby does it. These women may find that hand expressing works better for them, although this may not be the case all the time.

All of this aside, there are, of course, occasions where Mum just doesn't want to worry about expressing while away from her baby, and this is also okay. Things that can cause anxiety include:

- ◊ Taking the pump with her and storing it.
- ◊ Finding somewhere to express.
- ◊ Finding the time to express/missing out on part of the day to express.
- ◊ Storing the milk pumped.
- ◊ Asking for somewhere to express if needed, which can feel embarrassing.

It's important to remember that if your baby is used to being exclusively breastfed, then your breasts will likely become very full and sore while you are away, so you may need to express anyway. However, if you don't want to feed the milk you remove to your baby, you can hand express into a sink or during a shower until you feel less uncomfortably full.

I remember doing this myself while away at a breastfeeding conference. My son was 18 months old, and I hadn't expected my breasts to fill as he was only feeding two or three times a day. I was somewhat surprised to find myself hand expressing in the ladies' loos to ease my discomfort.

If a mother wishes for her baby to have formula while she is away, then it's a good idea to do a trial run to ensure that the baby takes the bottle, doesn't react badly to the formula, and to gauge how often Mum is likely to need to soften her breasts while away.

Some Things to be Aware of If You're Giving Bottles While Separated

◊ Your comfort. It is most likely that your breasts will fill and become uncomfortable if you don't use a pump to soften them often. How often will depend on how much your baby usually feeds?

◊ The baby may need extra reassurance in the form of cuddles and close contact with their carer while you are away. Remember that usually, all these needs are met at the breast.

◊ How and where you will express. Will you be staying in a hotel? If you're away with work, can they provide you with a private room to express in? Could you express in your car? Really take some time to consider when and where you may need to pump.

◊ Supply. If you are away for more than a day or two, particularly if your baby is young, then your supply may well reduce. This might be tricky to come back from. You could limit this risk by expressing several times each day while you are away.

◊ Breast refusal when you return. This sometimes happens if babies get used to a bottle while Mum is away and may also happen with toddlers or preschoolers who may have been close to weaning anyway. You can help to minimise the chances of this happening by ensuring lots of skin-to-skin contact once you return home and keeping things relaxed and calm, especially around offering your breast.

◊ Again, my experience of returning home after a night away was of having breasts full to bursting and expecting my little one to immediately want a feed. Instead, he just wanted to show me his new toy. It was a few hours before he latched. During that time, I stayed calm and remained nearby, waiting for him to ask to feed.

MAKING IT WORK FOR YOU

⬦ Look after your breasts as best you can while away. Consider options for milk removal if you are feeling very full.

⬦ Have the person looking after your baby use paced and responsive feeding methods, which may help to avoid bottle preference.

⬦ You could consider expressing in the days before you leave, so your baby has expressed milk while you are away.

⬦ Check if your baby will take a bottle or cup before you go.

⬦ Remember that the average baby not on solids needs around 750 – 900 ml of milk a day. You can divide that by how many times a day baby feeds to know how much is needed. For example, if your baby feeds eight times a day: 750 / 8 = 93.75 ml per feed, with up to 112.5 ml eight times a day being possible. Clearly you would round up or down a little for ease.

For When Mum is Exhausted and Needs a Break, So She Asks a Partner to Give a Bottle While She Goes to Sleep/Takes a Bath, etc.

Quick Glance Alternatives to Consider

⬦ Can Mum be supported to rest more in the day?

⬦ Are parents in a position to hire a cleaner, doula, or order a meal delivery service?

⬦ Can Mum find time for recharging between feeds?

⬦ Could the baby have Mum's expressed milk in a bottle?

"

The biggest benefit for me was that I could take a walk and then a shower every evening without worrying. My husband didn't even need to give a bottle very often, but on the few times he did, it was just an ounce to keep baby going until I was back.

~ Michelle

Why You Might Want to Combi-Feed

We live in a strange society where postnatal support for families seriously lacks in many ways. Let's consider Japan for a moment. There it is still expected that new mothers will stay indoors for at least the first month after the baby is born, with the tradition being 100 days after birth. Often, mums will return to their own mother's home during the last trimester and have access to her support during the early weeks after the baby is born. Here in the UK, and in much of the West, we might be fortunate enough to have family popping in to look after us. But it's unusual for us to have the level of support given by family in Japan and other cultures where the new mother is truly allowed the time and space she needs to heal.

This lack of support can mean that breastfeeding parents are dealing with the demands of a new baby *and* societal expectations regarding housework, nutrition, exercise, and socialising outside of the home. These mothers rarely have an opportunity to nap with the baby or to ask someone to help with many new-parent tasks. Mothers in the UK often tell me that they don't want to disturb their partner at night as he has to get up for work the next morning.

With all of this in mind, it is no surprise at all that many families choose to give the baby a bottle of formula at some point so that Mum can get some rest.

MAKING IT WORK

◊ Try to choose a time immediately after a breastfeed for Mum's break to begin. During the baby's fussy time is probably not the best opportunity. It can work better when you know the baby will be likely to sleep on another adult's chest for an hour or two.

◊ Be sure to use paced feeding responsively to avoid overfeeding and possible breast refusal later.

◊ Remember that your baby likely needs less milk than you think. Average intake after the first 4 weeks is 750 – 900 ml over 24 hours. So, if your baby feeds 8 times a day, then they need between 94 ml – 113 ml at a bottle feed (this is about 3 – 4 fl oz).

◊ If breasts begin to feel uncomfortable, the baby may want to feed if that is okay for Mum, or Mum could pump a little of her milk for comfort.

◊ If the top-ups are occasional–once a week or less–then supply is unlikely to be affected.

◊ If Mum is taking more frequent breaks, it can be helpful to try and make sure they happen at about the same time each day to avoid too much breast fullness.

Things to be Aware of

◊ You may inadvertently create more work if Mum needs to express her overly full, sore breasts.

◊ The baby may still want to breastfeed after the bottle.

◊ The baby may go longer than anticipated between the bottle and the next breastfeed, making engorgement and blocked ducts more likely.

◊ If a bottle is being given regularly, your supply will reduce. This may or may not be problematic, but it is less likely to cause issues if the bottle is given simultaneously (roughly) each day, and the same volume is given using a paced-feeding method.

Fear About Milk Supply During Growth Spurts

Quick Glance Alternatives to Consider

◊ Can you give your own expressed milk instead of formula?

◊ Find out about normal baby behaviour for reassurance.

◊ Remember the golden rules: heavy wet nappies, steady weight gain, baby happy after most feeds. If these are happening, the top-up almost certainly is not needed.

◊ Switch nurse and repeatedly swap breasts until the baby settles.

◊ Breast compressions to speed up milk flow.

Take your baby for a short walk or give them a bath and try again during fussy periods.

I panicked at every growth spurt even though people told me it was okay. Once I decided to give a couple of 60 ml bottles on those hard days, I relaxed, and I enjoyed breastfeeding a lot more.

~ Survey response

Why You Might Want to Combi-Feed

Babies often want to do a lot of feeding during growth spurts. This can be exhausting, and you may fear that your milk alone isn't enough. If you are thinking about combination-feeding because your baby has several hours in the evening or another part of the day where they are fussy and on and off the breast, then it can be helpful to know that this is usually normal behaviour. If your baby is gaining weight well, producing lots of wet and dirty nappies, and breastfeeding is comfortable for you, your milk is enough. You should also notice that for much of the day, breastfeeding is usually straightforward, with the baby happy to sleep in your arms or awake but content after feeding.

Babies cluster feed for all sorts of reasons, including, we think, to tank up on the small amounts of fat-rich milk present in softer breasts before they have a longer sleep. Cluster feeding may also help with milk supply. Frequent feeds keep prolactin levels high in your body, and prolactin is the hormone you use to make milk (Glasier, 1984). The more baby feeds, the more milk you will see in the coming days.

During a growth spurt, babies may need slightly more milk than usual, and cluster feeding might be because of this. As parents, we often worry about whether we are making enough milk during a growth spurt. Still, if we allow free access to the breast, even if it feels like that's a million feeds a day, then the baby will take what they need over the course of the day in nearly every single case. Your supply will go up to meet the new demand quickly as well—if you breastfeed frequently. People also often think that formula has more calories in it than breastmilk, so they believe that giving formula will somehow be more satisfying for the baby, but this just isn't true.

MAKING IT WORK

- ◊ Less is often more. You may find that just 20-30 ml, or 1 oz, give or take a little, will calm your baby enough for you to collect yourself before returning to breastfeeds.

- ◊ When giving small amounts of formula or breastmilk, a teaspoon or egg cup might help to avoid bottle preference.

- ◊ Try to offer the breast as much as you feel able. Remember that your baby needs extra nutrition now, and if you are usually exclusively breastfeeding then your body can make more to meet those needs.

- ◊ If your breasts feel full then either breastfeed or take a little milk off by expressing.

The Things to be Aware of if you Decide to Begin Combination-Feeding During a Growth Spurt

- ◊ The baby may go to the breast less than usual rather than more, as they naturally would during a growth spurt. This may reduce your supply and make more top-ups over a longer period more likely.

- ◊ Conversely, the baby may still want to breastfeed often. Frequent feeding is often about comfort and reassurance, as well as the nutrition.

- ◊ The baby may struggle to breastfeed. Some babies do decide they like the faster flow of a bottle and then might become agitated at the breast. This can lead to more top-ups and reduced supply over time (WHO, 1989).

> ◊ Your breast may become uncomfortably full, requiring you to express. Finding time to pump or hand express while the baby is fussy, and you are tired might feel extra challenging.

A Single Daily Bottle

When I surveyed infant feeding, this was the most common method of combination-feeding stated, with 47% of participants saying they gave one or two bottles a day. The next most common response was "several bottles a day," with 29% of responses indicating this. Let's take a look at some of the reasons for giving one bottle daily below.

Because It Seems to Lead to the Baby Sleeping Longer if Given at Night

Quick Glance Alternatives to Consider

- ◊ Bedsharing, if appropriate.
- ◊ Research normal baby sleep patterns for reassurance.
- ◊ Look into "sleep nudging" in books such as *The Gentle Sleep Book* by Sarah Ockwell Smith and *The No Cry Sleep Solution* by Elizabeth Pantley.

She maybe slept for an extra hour if we gave her formula at bedtime, sometimes less. To be honest this was like a miracle after the hourly wake ups!

~ Survey response

Why You Might Want to Combi-Feed

This is such an interesting topic. There seems to be a strong idea in our society that formula-fed babies sleep better and/or longer than breastfed babies. But where they are being fed an appropriate amount, the studies carried out on this topic tell us that actually formula-fed do wake less often than exclusively breastfed babies, but mothers of exclusively breastfed babies get significantly more sleep. This is because if you breastfeed at night, you can do so lying down and drift in and out of sleep. To formula-feed at night, you need to warm milk, sit up, and actively stay awake for the feed duration (Brown & Harries, 2015; Kendall-Tackett et al., 2011). In the Survey of Mothers' Sleep and Fatigue, a survey of 6,410 new mothers, mothers who exclusively breastfed and co-slept got by far the most sleep, followed by the exclusively breastfeeding, non-cosleeping mothers. Interestingly, the non-exclusively breastfeeding mothers who coslept got the least amount of sleep (Kendall-Tackett et al., 2015).

MAKING IT WORK

○ Try to be consistent with what time the bottle is offered. A good time can be when Mum is resting and someone else can step in for that feed. If you live alone or don't have much help, then right before you want to go bed could give a longer stretch of sleep (although this is not always true).

○ The first time you try, offer a little less milk than recommended, in case the baby reacts with a tummy ache.

○ Avoid overfeeding the baby to make them sleep longer. This may be dangerous. Paced bottle-feeds with smaller amounts of milk will help to avoid an overly full baby and potentially sore breasts from a missed feed.

Things to Be Aware of

○ Sometimes, people are tempted to give a big bottle of milk at night in the hope of making your baby sleep longer, but this practice may increase the risk of Sudden Infant Death Syndrome. They may also end up taking less milk overall at night, meaning they may not get as much nutrition as they need.

○ Not breastfeeding at all overnight might be hard on your milk supply, especially in the early weeks. Review the next section a little below this one about giving a bottle to help mums get more rest. This may work better for everyone than hoping the baby will sleep through the night before they are developmentally ready to do so.

○ The evidence we have does not suggest that formula-feeding will make a baby sleep longer.

For the Non-Breastfeeding Partner to Bond

Quick Glance Alternatives to Consider

○ Babywearing

○ Skin-to-skin contact

○ Bathing with the baby

○ Reading or singing to the baby

○ Baby massage

Daddy gave a bottle every evening at 6pm, and they both seemed to really enjoy it. I loved watching them gaze into each other's eyes.

~ Survey response

I discuss this in more depth in Chapter 8 but it is a common theme when I ask parents why they want to combination-feed. The idea that the non-breastfeeding parent wants or needs to feed a bottle to bond is long-standing, and certainly, many of the dads who do feed the baby occasionally say that they enjoy it. Mums also often say they enjoy watching their partner feed the baby as well (as the quote above demonstrates).

I do think it's important, though, to acknowledge that there are many, many other ways for parents to bond and help Mum. In fact, having the other parent feed a bottle may create more work for Mum if she also needs to express her full breasts a little later.

MAKING IT WORK

⬦ Try to limit the formula or expressed milk to once a day or less if possible. This will have less impact on milk supply.

⬦ Be consistent regarding the time a top-up is given.
A window of an hour or two will help your breasts to adjust.

⬦ Paced, responsive feeding with appropriate amounts is ideal (no more than around 3-4 fl oz once the baby is older than 4 weeks).

⬦ Express or breastfeed if breasts begin to feel uncomfortably full.

Things to Be Aware of

⬦ Mum may experience full, uncomfortable breasts.

⬦ Overfeeding may lead to more missed feeds.

⬦ Possibility of bottle preference.

⬦ Also, a possibility of bottle refusal in older babies.

⬦ The baby might be more likely to develop wind or colic when they have a bottle.

For Mum to Get a Reliable Chunk of Sleep Each Night

Quick Glance Alternatives to Consider

- Bedsharing, if appropriate
- Sidecar crib attached to the bed
- More rest for Mum in the day
- More help around the house
- An earlier bedtime for Mum

There were a handful of occasions in the first few months where I just needed to sleep. On those nights, my partner gave one bottle of expressed milk and then, if it was needed, a second bottle of formula. I usually woke up before that was needed because my boobs were full! Knowing I could have a night off sometimes definitely meant that I carried on breastfeeding for longer.

~ Jo

Why You Might Want to Combi-Feed

There's no doubt that becoming a new parent is often exhausting. We discussed the desire to give Mum a break a little earlier in the book, but this is more specific. I've occasionally supported families where the breastfeeding parent has an underlying medical condition where sleep becomes more important than it is for other people. For these families, if bedsharing isn't an appropriate or acceptable option, and formula is desired, then having the partner doing some night feeds is a logical way of ensuring Mum is well-rested. However, it is worth discussing how mums who breastfeed at night do seem to get a better quality of sleep than their bottle-feeding counterparts.

It is also important to figure out how to allow Mum some rest without compromising her milk supply. We know that going longer than six hours without breastfeeding means that prolactin levels drop to their baseline levels, so the message to make milk isn't as powerful. It may be that baby is breastfed at 9 pm or 10 pm. Someone else gives a bottle at the late evening feed. This means that Mum has had a good chunk of sleep by the time the baby wakes again somewhere in the early hours.

If the baby sleeps to a point where Mum is going longer than six hours without feeding, then reducing the supplement amount would be a good idea to ensure the baby is hungry a little sooner. Some mums may find that this is even a little too long. We all have our own storage capacity, and this varies between parents. Always be alert to how your body responds to a change and act accordingly. The simplest rule to remember is that if your breasts often feel uncomfortably full, you've probably gone a little too long and might want to try a smaller gap the next time you try.

MAKING IT WORK

◊ Ensure that any top-up feeds are offered consistently in a window of about two hours. This will help Mum's breasts to regulate faster.

◊ Try to avoid overfeeding the baby. A deep, prolonged sleep due to being too full is not considered safe for the baby, or Mum's breasts either. Around 3-4 fl oz is often recommended after the first four weeks of a baby's life.

Things to be Aware of

◊   Going long periods without feeding regularly will lead to a reduction in milk supply, and this is often more significant in the early weeks while supply is being established (Glasier, 1984). This might not be a problem if the bottle is being consistently offered at the same time each day, and the baby consistently sleeps for the same amount of time. However, it may become problematic over time. It's important to monitor milk supply the rest of the time to ensure the baby is happy at the breast and gaining weight well.

◊   Breasts may become full, increasing the risk of mastitis, blocked ducts, or breast abscesses. Breast fullness will improve over several days, and expressing to a comfortable level in the meantime will lower the risk of problems.

Mum Working Away from the Home for a Few Hours Each Day

Quick Glance Alternatives to Consider

◊   Flexible working – fewer hours per day, but more days per week.

◊   Temporary reduction of hours.

◊   Working from home.

◊   Having the baby brought to you for feeds.

◊   Returning home for feeds during an extended break.

◊   Expressed breast milk.

❝

I love breastfeeding, but I love my career and identity away from the home as well! When I returned to work, she was only 4 months old so needed lots of milk. I expressed once a day at lunchtime to keep myself comfortable and to provide her with some of my own milk, but the rest of the time she had formula when I was away, and I loved knowing she was happily and safely fed without me worrying about providing enough with a pump.

~ Alex

Why You Might Want to Combination-Feed

If the baby is taking solid food, this may not be an issue. If Mum is only away for two or three hours, then again, it may not be an issue. It is also surprising how often employers will be flexible enough to allow Mum to visit the baby for a feed during an extended lunch break, or even have the baby brought into the place of work for a breastfeed part-way through the day. However, if none of these scenarios are possible, then it stands to reason that your baby will need to be fed with a bottle or cup, either with expressed breastmilk or formula.

Things to Be Aware Of

○ If your baby solely relies on milk and you want to keep breastfeeding at home, then you will need to express to maintain supply while you are away. This may be as often as every three hours.

○ The baby might develop a bottle preference.

○ Milk supply may decrease, leading to more formula being given.

MAKING IT WORK

◊ Look at maternityaction.org for your rights under UK law.

◊ Take a pump to work with you or learn how to hand express so your breasts don't get too full during the first couple of weeks as they adjust to the change in demand.

◊ Talk to your employer about pumping breaks if you will need to remove milk.

◊ Ensure that whoever is looking after your baby can use paced, responsive feeding methods with appropriate amounts of expressed milk or formula.

Reassurance Following Early Weight Gain Concerns

Quick Glance Alternatives to Consider

◊ Speak to your healthcare provider about more frequent weight checks for reassurance.

◊ If weight gain is back on track, then consider weaning yourself off top-ups using some of the methods in Chapter 7.

It helped me to know I could just give a bottle whenever things felt overwhelming. I maybe did this every couple of weeks and it never affected my supply.

~ Jenny

Why You Might Want to Combination-Feed

When you have gone through the stress and fear of slow weight gain, it's not surprising that you may carry that fear with you going forward. You may want to keep one bottle a day to reassure yourself that the baby is getting enough milk. This situation might work well for everyone. If that's the case, then that's ideal.

If you would like to reduce or stop that one bottle, though, you can do this slowly so that you continue to be reassured that the baby is getting plenty from your breast. You would reduce the bottle by 10 ml only. After several days, try reducing it by another 10 ml. This could continue until the bottle is stopped altogether. If, at any point, you were worried about the baby being hungry, you would simply go back a step.

Things to Be Aware of

◊   Anxiety resulting from past experience may mean that you panic or worry whenever the baby wants to feed more often or becomes unsettled at the breast. This might lead to more top-ups being given and then a spiral into what we call the top-up trap. It's always important to keep an eye on the bigger picture with regard to weight gain, nappy count, and how the baby is **most** of the time.

◊   If the underlying reasons for slow weight gain were never addressed, it's possible that issues may pop up again further down the line and that a supplement each day has been masking the problem. Always seek good breastfeeding help if you have any worries about latching or how the baby is feeding.

MAKING IT WORK

○ Assuming good weight gain, try to limit top-ups to only when your baby is fussy at the breast, and try to give as little as you feel able to. Ten ml might be enough to help your baby focus on returning to the breast.

○ It may help to give supplements via a cup or spoon rather than a bottle if the volumes are small like this.

○ As always, use paced, responsive feeding. Your baby may not actually be hungry, but early experiences might lead to anxiety about changes in feeding patterns. Pacing feeds allows the baby to take control.

Gemma's Story

Gemma gave her baby formula for reassurance after some early challenges.

> I had an undiagnosed tongue-tie to contend with, despite asking again and again for professionals to help as I suspected it from day one.
>
> After high weight loss on day five, I was exhausted and sore and encouraged to express. Still, looking back, the advice on expressing wasn't good, and my daughter was borderline dehydrated and not settling at all (not sleeping, not settled/happy/content). I was stressed, so expressing was even harder. I felt like topping up with formula was the only option to make sure she got something, and immediately it became apparent that she wasn't getting much from me at all because 5 ml of formula knocked her out.
>
> I eventually had a consultation with an IBCLC because I just didn't feel like I was getting anywhere with BF despite being pretty well-read on it, and after a full consult, she diagnosed an obvious TT, which I then had corrected privately at 1-month-old.

I then had a course of domperidone that I had researched myself. My GP and the doctor who fixed the tongue-tie agreed I should take it to try and bring my milk back up, as, by this point, she had been getting very little from me at all. It was very successful.

It all improved a lot after that very difficult start, but by that point, my mental health had taken a battering. I ended up combination-feeding to make sure I had some relief, that my husband could still take over a bit when I needed him to. It worked very well, but I felt like this was completely driven by me, and the team at the hospital and community midwives weren't interested in supporting me to combination-feed.

I kind of understand because you get the best and worst of both sides. But I'm still glad we did it! We combination-fed to nearly 19 months, when I decided that it was a good time for us to stop, which, although I know was the right decision, I still feel guilty about, and she's now 3.5!

Simple Parental Preference!

I always said I wanted to use bottles and breast and I wish there was more support for me. Once we figured out how to get the balance right, we were able to breastfeed until my baby was over 2 years old.

~ Ellie

It's so important to acknowledge that sometimes families choose combi-feeding. There can be many reasons for this, from plain preference to experiencing aversion or Dysphoric Milk- Ejection Reflex, commonly called D-MER, or in some cases, a history of abuse in Mum's life. If everyone is comfortable with the arrangement, then there's no reason to change what you are doing.

Things to Be Aware of

◊ Giving a bottle daily may make it more likely that you give more bottles any time your baby behaves differently at the breast. Normal growth spurt behaviour or illness could make you worry about your milk supply. Giving more formula at this point could reduce your supply, meaning that the new top-up becomes required.

◊ Daily bottles may make it more likely that the baby prefers the flow of a bottle over the breast, particularly when the breast is softer and flowing more slowly at certain times of the day or at the end of a feed.

Several Bottles Each Day

In my survey, almost 30% of families indicated that they gave several bottles a day, and the biggest reason for this was slow weight gain when exclusively breastfeeding. We will look at this and other reasons below.

MAKING IT WORK

◊ Try to be consistent with the number of bottle feeds per day or week, and with the time of day these top-ups are given.

◊ Remember: paced, responsive feeding in appropriate amounts is key!

Baby Struggles to Gain Weight as Needed When Exclusively Breastfed

Quick Glance Alternatives to Consider

◊ An at-breast supplementing system

◊ Donor milk

◊ Prescription or herbal galactagogues if safe and appropriate

◊ Expressed milk

"

"I cannot describe the relief when I realised I could carry on breastfeeding and help my baby to grow with just 20 mls of formula a few times a day."

~ Survey response

There is lots of practical information for overcoming low milk supply or poor milk transfer in Chapter 6. What I want to say in this section, though, is that mixed feeding due to slow weight gain is quite common. The causes for slow weight gain are often a mix of the baby not latching as well as they could be (so removing less milk than is needed, leading to a supply reduction) and spiralling weight concerns.

Many parents feel guilty or a sense of failure when formula is medically indicated. I know this is a tough experience to deal with. Remember that we believe there are three million germ-killing cells in every teaspoon of breastmilk. Combination-feeding in this situation is not pointless or a failure on your part as a mother. The formula can be given as if it's a medicine until you can resolve the issues that led to the bottles needing to be introduced. Look at Chapter 4 for information on low-supply causes and how to get support, and Chapter 6 for galactagogues.

Things to Be Aware of

⬧ Giving formula while not expressing to maintain or build milk supply will only lead to less breastmilk being made.

⬧ Seeking good support to help you with the underlying causes is important if you want to return to exclusive breastfeeding.

⬧ Feelings of grief when breastfeeding doesn't go to plan are common. You might want to talk your feelings through with a breastfeeding trained supporter such as a breastfeeding counsellor.

> ## MAKING IT WORK
>
> ◊ Small volumes of top-up after breastfeeds are often most helpful as they avoid overfilling your baby, so the next breastfeed is less likely to be delayed by a full tummy.
>
> ◊ While it is often advised to limit feeds to Mum and one other person, in the case of topping up for weight worries, expanding the number of helpers a little can help free up time for Mum to pump, if a return to exclusive breastfeeding is desired.

Breastfeeding is Painful

Quick Glance Alternatives to Consider

◊ Find excellent, highly skilled breastfeeding support. This may not be accessible as a standard breastfeeding support option in your area.

◊ If it's a case of reducing breastfeeding against your preference, then consider nipple shields, ideally with good breastfeeding support. You need to be sure that the shield you choose fits you well and that you follow the instructions for applying it properly. The manufacturers have information regarding both on their websites.

Consider expressing and feeding your baby your milk via a cup or bottle instead of formula top-ups.

"I just needed a break from the pain. I gave bottles several times in those first 3 weeks. Because of good support to manage this from an IBCLC, I was able to return to full breastfeeding once we got the tongue-tie cut."

~ Martha

When breastfeeding is painful, many mothers find themselves dreading every feed, and formula quickly begins to feel like an option for giving sore nipples a breather. If this is the preferred choice, then try to express to maintain your milk supply if you are giving formula regularly. A one-off bottle a couple of days a week won't usually hurt milk supply, but if you are looking to give several feeds a day over several days this way, then expressing will help you to keep your supply normal when you are ready to return to breastfeeding. Of course, if after a few days of combination-feeding, you decide you prefer to bottle feed, then you can ease off on the expressing until your milk dries up.

Things to Be Aware of

◊ Simply giving a bottle won't address the underlying cause of your pain and may make latching even more challenging.

◊ You may need to express if you want to return to exclusive breastfeeding, so giving your own milk, pumped, might be a cheaper and more sustainable option.

> ## MAKING IT WORK
>
> ◊ If your goal is to return to breastfeeding exclusively, then limit bottles to as few as you can stand.
>
> ◊ If feeding is too painful but you don't want to stop, then expressing each breast at least 8 times a day for 15 to 20 minutes will help to maintain supply while you work on your challenges.
>
> ◊ As always, paced, responsive feedings are recommended, especially for newborns who don't necessarily need a specified amount per feed.

Mum Prefers the Flexibility of Knowing She Can Leave Her Baby with Someone Else

Quick Glance Alternatives to Consider

◊ Babies are often welcome anywhere and are surprisingly good at sleeping in strange, noisy places.

◊ Can outings be shorter, so they happen between breastfeeds?

◊ With regard to hospital stays, often, a carer will be permitted to bring your baby onto the ward for feedings. You would need to talk to the hospital for confirmation of this.

◊ Expressed breastmilk can allow you some time away.

"I was in and out of hospital and one thing I never had to worry about was whether my baby would take a bottle."

~ Survey response

It's easy to think that all breastfeeding parents want to be very close to their babies day and night for several months. While this does apply to many mothers, there are some who need a little bit of time and headspace alone for their own mental health. Other scenarios where Mum may need the baby to take a bottle include if she needs to have surgery or is caring for a sick or elderly relative where she is called away at short notice to provide support. She may have other children with additional needs or have a long-term health condition, which means she struggles to care for her baby at times. In all these cases, it makes sense that we know the baby will take nutrition from another source. For information on helping the baby take a bottle, see Chapter 7.

Things to Be Aware of

◊ Breast fullness can potentially lead to blocked ducts or mastitis.

◊ The baby may refuse to take the bottle.

◊ Reduced milk supply if separation is prolonged.

◊ Breast refusal upon Mum's return if separation is prolonged.

◊ Once again, simple parental preference.

MAKING IT WORK

◊ It may be helpful to offer the baby a bottle a couple of times a week to reduce the chances of bottle refusal.

◊ Remember that you may need to express if you will be away for more than a few hours and your breasts become full.

◊ Paced, responsive feeds of appropriate volumes are the most important thing to consider.

For Comfort Where a Baby is Mostly Formula-fed

Quick Glance Alternatives to Consider

- Use an at-breast supplementing device.
- Even if your baby is receiving all their nutrition from a bottle, you can still enjoy the other aspects of breastfeeding as long as the baby will latch. Remember that the breast is the natural place for babies to find comfort, reassurance, pain relief, and support falling asleep.

It helped to heal me. Breastfeeding wasn't happening but I was taught the words 'breast nurturing,' and that was exactly what we did.

~ Louise

Things to Be Aware of

- As supply dwindles, the baby may refuse to latch.
- If the baby latches often, milk supply may increase.
- Even tiny amounts of breastmilk have been demonstrated to be beneficial to babies.

MAKING IT WORK FOR YOU

- Try offering the breast during skin-to-skin time or after a bottle feed.
- Enjoy it!

During Relactation

Relactation is the process of rebuilding a milk supply after a period of not breastfeeding. It is often carried out for the same baby, for an adopted baby, or as part of a co-breastfeeding relationship where both partners want to breastfeed.

The first time he latched I felt the rush of love everyone kept talking about.

~ Lucy

Things to Be Aware of

◊ Latching may not happen until your milk supply has begun to rebuild. As you can see, there are many reasons for combination-feeding, and there is no judgement here regarding any of them. Breastfeeding can take many forms, and any breastfeeding is beneficial to the baby and mum.

MAKING IT WORK FOR YOU

◊ Take it slowly and consider working with a skilled breastfeeding supporter to support latching, perhaps with at-breast supplementing via a feeding tube taped to the breast, or with a nipple shield.

Potential Problems with Combination-Feeding (and Some Ways to Limit Them)

I think it's important to be aware that, while combination-feeding works well for lots of families, there are some possible pitfalls to know about.

◊ The baby may struggle to switch between breast and bottle. There is some anecdotal evidence, and a general theory that paced bottle-feeding will help to avoid what is sometimes called bottle preference or nipple confusion.

◊ You may be at greater risk of mastitis, at least initially. Keeping an eye on your breasts and expressing a little milk or breastfeeding when they feel full can reduce this risk.

◊ The baby might be allergic to the formula. While it is true that some babies show allergic reactions to cow's milk protein through Mum's milk, this is often much more obvious and unpleasant if the baby is exposed to cow's milk directly from formula (Host et al., 1988). You could talk to your doctor about a prescription formula milk instead, return to full breastfeeding, or research informal milk donation from other breastfeeding parents.

◊ Your baby might not accept a bottle. You could offer a cup instead. You may also find that persistent, gentle offering of the bottle does eventually lead to acceptance. Tips for encouraging baby to take a bottle include trying warmer or cooler milk than usual, trying different bottle types, having a different person try, and turning baby away from the caregiver while feeding (just while baby gets used to the bottle – always have them facing the carer again once baby is relaxed and comfortable).

◊ Your supply might reduce more than you wanted it to, particularly if the formula makes your baby sleep longer than usual. Try to pace bottle feeds to avoid overfeeding and add in more breastfeeds if you feel that your supply is getting too low. You could express if you didn't want to offer the breast more often. You can find instructions for paced feeding further on in the book.

The top-up trap. This is an important issue to talk about. The top-up trap is where you begin by giving a single top-up, perhaps out of fear that you don't have enough milk or because you need to be separated. The baby may gulp down that bottle, confirming your fear that your own milk isn't good enough. Then, because it's easier to overfeed a baby with the bottle and because formula is slower to be digested, you may find that your baby goes longer than usual before they want another breastfeed. In the meantime, your breasts fill up, which tells your body to make *less* milk.

While this isn't usually a big problem with occasional bottles, if you're giving more frequent supplements, then your supply will reduce. A reduced supply might mean that your baby is fussy at the breast, which makes you worry more, so you give more top-ups. The more top-ups you give, the more your baby wants to bottle-feed, the less you feed at the breast, and the lower your supply gets.

Following the guidelines in this book will help you avoid this situation, and you can read the chapter on breastmilk to understand how milk production works. It is absolutely the case that knowledge is power here, and once you know what might happen and why you are less likely to fall into the top-up trap.

⚠ Why Is Exclusive Breastfeeding Recommended?

This is a section that might feel uncomfortable or difficult to read, but it's also a section that was conspicuous by its omission in early drafts of this book. I discuss the risks of formula in the next chapter, but I don't discuss the reasons why exclusive breastfeeding is recommended all over the world. I'll discuss these reasons a little below, but as with the formula risks, please do skip this section if you are not in the right frame of mind to read it. This book is here to help, not to trigger difficult feelings.

The introduction of formula to babies seems to alter their gut flora, and we are still researching the immunological effects of this. Human stomachs are designed to receive human milk, which is made just for human babies. Cow's milk, even if it has been modified, is not the same as human milk, and we know that it does lead to changes in the baby's gut. The proteins are different as well.

Formula doesn't contain the live elements of breastmilk, and it doesn't adapt according to the environment. There is some evidence that suggests that babies given formula in the early days of life may be more likely to develop allergies because breastmilk coats the digestive tract, but formula falls through the cell gaps there. While we might not be completely sure of the long-term effects of all these little things, we do know that the biological norm is altered with the introduction of small amounts of formula.

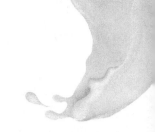

CHAPTER 3

All About Formula

Formula is a fascinating topic. If we're going to be spending a lot of time talking about how and when it's used for combination-feeding, it seems sensible to take a look at its history, its nutritional make-up, and how to prepare and store it.

History

Up until the 19th century, if a mother couldn't breastfeed, then the best and most common alternative was to employ a wet nurse. Wet-nursing dates back as at least 2000 BC and has probably been going on for as long as humans existed. The practice is still around today, albeit with a lot more stigma surrounding it. The Old Testament (Book of Exodus) describes the need for baby Moses to have a wet nurse.

The history is interesting, and, at times, heart-breaking. Enslaved wet nurses, for example, were often expected to breastfeed the slave owner's babies over and above their own. In the Victorian Era, baby farming was a practice where people would be paid to take in babies and feed them. Tragically, these babies often died as their care was held as secondary to the income they brought in. However, for a long time, wet-nursing was respectable, and pay disputes involving wet nurses have even been documented in ancient Rome. Ancient physicians would have long lists of what mothers should look for when choosing a nurse. And of course, it was an honour to be a wet nurse for royalty.

It also seems that babies were fed with animal milk in ancient times. Containers found in infant graves have been found to have traces of animal casein in them. This fact, combined with the presence of a crude teat or spout, tells us that these babies likely died due to unhygienic feeding practices or simply through malnutrition from being fed on inappropriate milk alternatives.

Feeding devices were also problematic. By the beginning of the 19th century, around one-third of babies fed away from the breast were dying. In a similar vein, it was common to "hand feed" cows' milk to babies in Norway in the 1600s and 1700s. This was so deadly that women would often have 30 pregnancies because so many of the babies would die as a result of not being breastfed (Hastrup, 1992).

In 1865, a chemist called Justus von Liebig developed, patented, and then started to market an infant food. Liebig's formula was made from cow's milk, wheat and malt flour, and potassium bicarbonate. It was widely considered to be the perfect food for babies (Radbill, 1981).

In 1810, Nicholas Appert found a way to sterilise food and keep it in sealed containers. This invention was followed by the creation of evaporated milk, which was patented in 1835 by a man called William Newton. In 1853, Texan Gale Borden added sugar to this evaporated milk and called it Condensed Milk. It soon became a popular food for babies. John B. Myerling then developed an unsweetened condensed milk in 1885 and called it evaporated milk. Myerling's milk was often recommended by paediatricians in the 1930s and 1940s as a way to feed babies (Radbill, 1981).

Plenty of formulas were quickly introduced after Liebig's infant food and the invention of evaporated milk. In 1883, there were 27 brands of infant food (Fomon, 2001). These came in a powdered form and included carbohydrates like sugar and starch. Brands for these milks and foods included Nestlé's Food®, Horlick's Malted Milk®, Hill's Malted Biscuit Powder®, and Robinson's Patent Barley®. The foods were high in fat, but they didn't have many of the important nutrients such as protein, vitamins, and minerals. As time went on, these foods did improve and began to contain more nutrients.

Formula was associated with many infant deaths, particularly during the warmer summer months (Wickes, 1953) because milk left in bottles would quickly go bad (Weinberg, 1993). Between 1890 and 1910, people began to realise the importance of cleanliness and made several improvements to hygiene around formula and bottles. Improvements included the introduction of milk clinics to provide clean milk to the public (Greer & Apple, 1991). By 1912, rubber nipples that were easy to clean were thankfully available, and many homes could keep milk safely in an icebox.

Amazingly, advertising wasn't regulated until the 1930s. Formula companies could say anything they liked to both doctors and the public. By the 1940s, infant formula was considered normal and safe by both the public and the medical profession. Both breastfeeding rates dropped consistently until the 1970s.

In the 1980s, the World Health Organisation (WHO) stepped in. They were seeing underhand marketing practices by the formula companies, leading to the deaths of millions of babies worldwide, especially in developing countries. One of the issues was that the formula sellers were telling mothers and their medical professionals that the women couldn't make good enough milk for their babies. The hospitals were then sending families home with free samples of formula. This was thanks to the formula reps having access to both parents and hospital staff.

Mums would feed the baby the formula, often believing it was better than their own milk. Then their milk supply would decrease, and once the sample ran out, she would be forced to buy more. Often, they couldn't afford to do this, so they would water the formula down to stretch it, or they would make it with cold water due to no electricity supply.

In developing countries, water was often dirty and needed to be fetched from a shared local water source. Other family members would go without good nutrition to ensure that the baby was fed with the required formula milk. Babies died from malnutrition or contaminated milk.

All of this was preventable by simply removing the sales reps from birth and postnatal spaces, ensuring ethical practices from the companies responsible, and providing breastfeeding education to medical professionals that was not influenced, sponsored, or provided by the formula industry. (Sadly, this is still not guaranteed, and a big part of UK formula influence comes from industry-sponsored training.)

The WHO developed their International Code for the Marketing of Breastmilk Substitutes in 1981 (The Code). Since then, although there has been more regulation of formula companies, the Code is not compulsory for countries to sign up to. As a result, it may only be partially applied (as in the UK), maybe poorly implemented or monitored, and the companies are not well known for adhering to the Code as well as they are supposed to.

A general misunderstanding from the public as to why the Code exists also leads to people assuming its aim is to force people to breastfeed, or to punish them for not breastfeeding. This means that contraventions are not reported or even noticed a lot of the time.

To clear up possible confusion, the Code states the following:

◊ There may be no advertising of the products covered by the Code to the public.

◊ Free samples cannot be given to parents.

◊ Healthcare facilities cannot advertise the products covered.

◊ Formula companies can't employ "nurses" or parentcraft workers to support parents.

◊ Formula companies cannot give gifts or personal samples to people working in healthcare.

◊ There should not be any words or pictures that idealise bottle-feeding on the products being sold.

- ⬦ Information given to health workers should be scientific and factual.

- ⬦ All labels should explain the risks of formula-feeding, as well as the costs and hazards associated with this.

- ⬦ Products not safe for babies must not be advertised for babies (for example, condensed milk).

- ⬦ All products must be high quality and suitable for storage in the country of use.

None of these guidelines are there to make life harder for formula-feeding families. They exist to protect those using the products covered by the Code. As an example, if formula was allowed to be placed on special offer, mums worried about their milk supply are more likely to buy it, and then may find that their supply drops more if they feed the formula without expressing/seeking support. Once the formula is no longer on offer, it becomes expensive for her to buy.

Another reason formula shouldn't be marked down as an incentive to buy it is because all the companies do to make up for this lost income is make their other products more expensive. They become less accessible to those who need them. The only winner here is the company.

Formula and the Environment

I am aware that some people reading this book will be keen to know what impact formula-feeding has on the environment, and how you may be able to reduce that impact. I will list some of the concerns below and some ideas for improving the situation where you can. Please always remember, though, that if you are giving any breastmilk, you are reducing the impact on the environment.

I want to first acknowledge that we can talk about the environment all we like, but we can't place blame on families. Until the manufacture, transport, and storage of products become more environmentally friendly, all we can do is firefight the situation. Industry has a far, far bigger impact on the environment than any one person or household ever can.

◇ Waste from formula packaging, bottle, and teats.

Items such as formula tins, bottles, or cartons, teats, and feeding bottles tend to find their way into landfill. The waste from the tins alone equates to 150 million tins for every million babies who are exclusively formula-fed. This can be broken down into 23,333 tons of metal and 336 tons of waste from the paper labels (Radford, 1991).

We, thankfully, have better recycling facilities than ever before, so using these for as much of your waste as possible will help. You can buy glass feeding bottles now, rather than plastic, which may be kinder to the planet and your baby. You could also use a cup to feed the baby if you are giving small amounts of top-ups. There are further methods to consider as well, including using a teaspoon or an at breast supplementing device.

Every time you breastfeed, you reduce the amount going into landfill. Let's imagine the average baby gets through one tin of formula a week if they are only being formula-fed. If you are feeding your baby 50% at the breast, you will save over 20 tins being sent to landfill in a year. If you are providing ¾ breastmilk, that's over 30 tins not adding to the problem.

On a similar note, let's imagine you use six cartons of formula a day for an exclusively bottle-fed baby. Just 50% breastfeeding will keep 21 cartons out of your bin every single week!

While bottled or cartons of formula are increasingly recommended for newborns, the powdered formula does create a lot less waste in terms of landfill, and the tins can often be reused for household storage, plant pots, or stacking toys for toddlers.

◊ **More period products ending up in landfills due to an earlier return of your cycle.**

Women who exclusively breastfeed often see a delay in their monthly period returning, usually for at least six months, but often for a year or more. Once the baby is no longer exclusively breastfed, it becomes likely that your periods will return, meaning you will need to use menstruation products. If you are using single-use items for your period, you will be contributing to the vast number that ends up in landfill each year.

This is, thankfully, a fairly easy issue to overcome in our modern world. Many period products are eco-friendly now, including cloth pads, reusable cups, and period underwear.

◊ **The dairy industry.**

As the daughter of a farmer, I remember the shock I felt at learning about how the global dairy industry has a negative impact on the environment. The dairy industry currently makes up about 30% of Global Greenhouse Emissions. For every 100 g of raw milk produced, about 20% of that is used to make formula.

Another issue is the amount of water required for the safe running of the dairy industry. We need to consider that cows drink a lot of water, and a lot more is used for cleaning the yard, milking parlour, and milk tanks. It's been estimated that it takes 4,700 litres of milk to produce one kilogram of infant milk powder.

An exclusively formula-fed baby will use around 57 kg of milk powder in the first two years of life according to Mathilde Cohen and Yoriko Otomo (2017). Remember that every breastfeed you provide your baby reduces that impact. Every single feed helps.

For a more in-depth look at the impact of formula-feeding on the environment, I highly recommend the book *The Politics of Breastfeeding* by Gabrielle Palmer.

Formula vs Breastfeeding Controversy

Look on any social media or parenting forum, and you will soon find controversy around infant feeding. There are entire groups and pages dedicated to attacking either formula or breastfeeding, depending on which "side" the proponents fall into. Breastfeeding workers are at times called "lactivists," or even "Nazis." Formula-feeding mums are called desperate formula-feeders (DFF) or "ignorant." Both sides are guilty at times of falsely and horribly accusing the other of abusing their children. Both sides contribute negatively to the way breastfeeding is portrayed in our world.

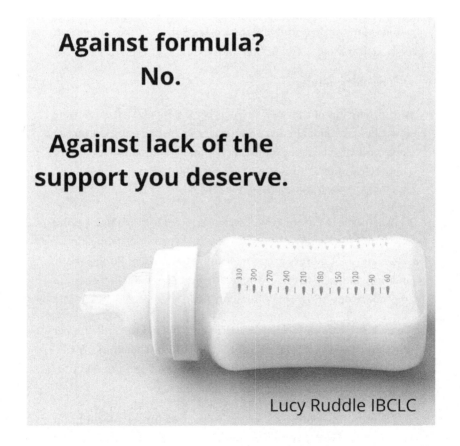

Against formula?
No.

Against lack of the support you deserve.

Lucy Ruddle IBCLC

The controversy and anger are often rooted in guilt of some kind and a lack of awareness regarding individual circumstances. Of course, there's the relative safety of a computer screen providing a degree of anonymity for the attacker. Fortunately, most of the public understands that these hate pages are not the norm and are not helpful for anyone.

If you believe formula is the invention of the devil, you will avoid using it, even if it's medically indicated. If you believe breastfeeders are smug hippies, hellbent on forcing you to exclusively breastfeed, then you won't reach out to them if you want help to provide breastmilk to your baby, in whatever quantity. It makes no sense for us, as sensible adults, to essentially sling mud at each other for feeding our babies.

There's a deeper problem here than women throwing hurtful words at each other across the Internet. The anger and strong opinions that infant feeding brings up are good at shutting down sensible discussion. This results in formula-feeding mums not knowing how to prepare formula safely and breastfeeding mums, not understanding what abnormal breastfeeding behaviour needing additional calories looks like.

No one is informed in the best possible way. Everyone ends up in an echo chamber, which is incredibly detrimental to parents and their babies. Mothers need support, information, and understanding. The Internet can be amazing at that, but it can also be a logistical nightmare.

Of course, part of the issue for such controversy stems from the way research into the field of infant feeding pulls on parental guilt. Studies discussing the risks of formula, such as an increased likelihood of Sudden Infant Death Syndrome, gastroenteritis, pneumonia, diabetes, and leukaemia (Stuebe, 2009), often upset parents for several reasons. We all want to do what's best for our babies, and hearing that the way you fed your baby might have increased the chances of that baby becoming sick might make us feel that we're being called bad parents.

Defensiveness is a natural response to hearing something that makes us feel uncomfortable. Our brains are wired to try to protect us in this way. Recognising the defensive feelings of anger or shame, labelling those feelings, and then just sitting with them for a while can be helpful as we begin to digest new information.

One question I try to always ask myself when I find myself angry at someone else's statement is: "What is the situation like from this person's perspective?" I find it effective for calming myself down and accessing the empathy, which allows me to refocus and learn something new. Perhaps this is something we could all try to practice: empathy and understanding for each other, rather than accusations.

We might not resonate with what is being said in the research about infant feeding because our children and ourselves were formula-fed and are healthy. Indeed, many of the studies are inconclusive or contradict each other. The headlines, and the way the studies are discussed, can also feel confrontational and cold.

It's important to keep in mind the voices of the majority of women when we are considering how we personally feel. Eighty-one percent say they wanted to breastfeed for longer in the UK. People are stopping breastfeeding because they didn't feel able to continue, not because they were ready to stop. When asked why they wanted to continue, most can say that "breastfeeding is better for the baby."

Mothers don't stop doing something they see as important for their babies because they are ignorant or lazy. They stopped, by and large, because they didn't have the support they needed. They stopped because often, no one even knows what that good support should look like, never mind that it's missing.

The problem is that because so many people don't understand what outstanding breastfeeding support looks like, they don't know that kind of support existed, and they could have accessed it. They may get angry when breastfeeding supporters point out that better help might have resulted in a different outcome. Then, breastfeeding supporters assume that this anger is defensiveness and denial, and everyone ends up mad at everyone else. It is the perfect example of a society pitching women against women rather than supporting them to lift each other up.

Why is any of this relevant in a book about combination-feeding? Well, I'd very much like to live in a world where a few things happen automatically.

1.   Parents have access to parent-focused, empathic, and highly skilled evidence-based lactation support as default.

2.   We are open and clear about why breastfeeding is important and lovely, and everyone has easy access to this information from childhood.

3.   For those who are sure they don't want to or can't breastfeed, there is no judgement, but instead, there is solid, clear information and evidence-based support.

The more controversy we allow to bubble up in unkind words, the harder it becomes to feed our babies in *any* way without feeling guilty for something. If we could just all be honest and supportive at the same time, there would be less guilt, anger, and defence – and a lot more parental confidence and empathy for everyone.

Choosing a Formula

Choosing an infant formula:

Whilst it appears that there is a huge range of infant formula available, most babies only need what is usually called a "first" infant formula if they are mixed fed or formula fed in the first year of life. Whilst different brands might suggest that they are superiour in some way or another, all infant formula marketed in the UK must meed the same regulations for ingredients. In the past companies were allowed to advertise their milks as "being closer to breastmilk" but it has been against the law to compare breastmilk with infant formula since 2007 as infant formula can only provide the nutrients a baby needs and cannot mimic the many live and unique ingredients which protect infants from infection or illness. Some infant formula make statements that their product is easier to digest or can prevent colic or constipation, but babies are able to digest proteins in milk and evidence for these benefits have not been agreed by scientific bodies in the UK.

It is important to remember that if an ingredient you could add to infant formula has been proven to offer a health benefit for baby, then ALL infant formulas would be required to include it under UK law. So, what is the best way to choose a formula? You may decide that organic ingredients are important to you and want to choose one of the organic infant formula, or else you may just want to choose one which is readily available in your nearest shop and which you can afford.

Ingredients

The European Commission has defined a set of rules for the ingredients. Formula needs to provide to meet all of a baby's nutritional needs during the first year. The ingredients below must be included.

You may also want to look at the list of breastmilk ingredients discussed later on in this book. That list is a lot longer. When combination-feeding, you are still giving your baby all of the amazing ingredients found in your breastmilk, with formula providing some extra in the form of nutrition.

Vitamin D is important to mention here too. Sometimes people are confused about why breastfed babies are required to take vitamin D supplements, but formula-fed babies are not. In the Northern Hemisphere, many of us, including adults, are deficient in vitamin D, which is a "sunshine" vitamin, not a "food" vitamin. The NHS in the UK recommends that everyone takes vitamin D. Babies do absorb the vitamin D present in breastmilk better than in formula so that you will find high amounts in infant milks compared to vitamin drops. This is to ensure formula-fed babies get enough.

Protein

Protein is important for growth, neurodevelopment and hormonal regulation.

Fat

Fat is important for babies and makes up about 50% of their daily calorie intake. Fat helps the body to absorb vitamins A, D,

E, and K, and it is essential for neurological development and brain function.

Vitamins and Minerals

Vitamin C supports the immune system and helps the body to absorb Iron.

Vitamin A is important for supporting the immune system and for vision and healthy skin.

Vitamin D supports the growth of bones and muscles.

Vitamin E supports the immune system and protects the eyes and skin.

Vitamin K is needed for blood clotting.

B1 is used for turning food into energy.

B2 keeps the eyes and nervous system healthy.

B6 makes haemoglobin, the substance in red blood cells that carries oxygen through the body.

B12 makes red blood cells and helps the body absorb folic acid.

Calcium supports bone, teeth and heart strength, and aids in blood clotting

Phosphorous helps the body to use carbohydrates and fat as well as helping to form bones and teeth.

Magnesium helps with muscle and nerve function, as well as the formation of DNA

Iron is important for oxygen transportation around the body

Zinc helps to support the immune system

Manganese is important for many chemical and metabolic processes in the body

Copper does lots of things including helping to form red blood cells and maintain nerves, healthy bones and immune function.

Iodine makes thyroid hormones

Sodium helps to maintain normal blood pressure

Potassium helps to maintain fluid balance.

Chloride helps to balance fluid and blood volume.

Anti-Reflux Milks

If you think your baby has reflux, then this should be diagnosed by your GP. Many babies posset after feeds or seem squirmy, but this is rarely actually a problem for them. Anti-reflux milks in the UK don't have to follow the same compositional and labelling requirements as other infant formulas, so they should only be used under medical supervision. Anti-reflux milks are often thickened with things like potato starch or locust bean gum, and manufacturers recommend that the powder is added to water at a lower temperature than is needed to kill any bacteria in the powder. Anti-reflux milks may also be contraindicated with some medications.

Soya-Protein-Based Formula

Despite being found in supermarkets, Soya-protein formula is not recommended for babies in the first 6 months of life in the UK unless medically recommended. There are concerns that the phyto-oestrogens in soya may impact sexual maturation of infants and that sugars present may damage developing teeth.

As of June 2020, there are no infant formulas on the UK market that are suitable for vegans, but it is likely that these may be available in the future. Although soy formula is not made from animal milk, the vitamin D used is sourced from the lanolin in sheep's wool, and this formula is not recommended in the first six months of life.

Goats' Milk-Based Formula

There are a number of infant formulas that are made from goats' rather than cows' milk. They may claim to be softer on the baby's tummy or easily digested/better tolerated than cow's milk formula, but there is no evidence to support this claim. All infant formula must have the same protein composition regardless of whether they are based on cows' or goats' milk. These infant formulas are not less allergenic than cows' milk-based infant formula, and if there are concerns about a food allergy, then this should be discussed with a health visitor or GP.

Homemade Formula

Alarmingly you can find recipes online for homemade infant formula – more commonly in the U. S. than in the UK. Making your own formula is risky and potentially dangerous. As this is an issue found a lot more in the States, I was only able to find statements from organisations in America, but it's fair to say that the same type of concern does apply in the UK, where parents do occasionally ask about making their own formula at home. The American Academy of Paediatrics is clear on its stance here, telling us that homemade formula will likely have either not enough of the right nutrients, or too many, which can be dangerous. Even a few days of homemade formula could have awful, lasting results. The Food and Drug Administration, also in America, takes the same line as the AAP stating categorically that they do not recommend home made formula due to the significant risk of error in combining the ingredients.

A 2020 study looked at the different places online where you could read how to make your own formula. They state: "76.3% and 20.3% either advertised or sold ingredients or recipe kits respectively." Basically, most of them were able to make profit from parents making their own formula. The thing which might be most alarming about this study was that out of the 59 blogs included, only 7 claimed that the writer was a nutritionist (Davis, Knol, Crowe-White, Turner, & McKinley, 2020).

Breastfeeding is rarely unsafe even when an allergy is suspected or diagnosed. Support to continue breastfeeding can be found locally or via the national helplines. Where possible and appropriate, you might prefer to consider exclusive breastfeeding or the use of peer-to-peer-sourced donor milk instead of a prescription formula.

Prescription Formula

There are several conditions that require a specialist infant formula, and if your baby is diagnosed with one of these, a specialist formula will be prescribed. The most common reason for the use of a specialist formula is if a baby is allergic to cows' milk. While continued breastfeeding is recommended if a baby is diagnosed with a cows' milk allergy, support will be given with an appropriate infant milk if the baby is fully or partially formula-fed.

For most babies with a cows' milk allergy, an extensively hydrolysed formula (eHF) is safe. For babies with more complex food allergies, an amino acid-based formula is recommended.

Stage-2 Milk

Follow-on formula, also called Stage-2 milks, are marketed for babies aged 6-12 months and older. There is no need for infants to move on to follow on formula after six months, and these milks are not recommended by health bodies in the UK. There is plenty of iron in first infant formula to meet the needs of older babies alongside solid foods, and it is important that babies are introduced to a range of varied foods in the second 6 months of life so they can start to meet their nutritional needs from food rather than milk alone.

Children over the age of one who are not having breastmilk can usually move on to whole animal milk as their main milk drink and do not need toddler growing-up milks. If desired, some plant milks are suitable instead of dairy products, including oat and soya milk.

Volumes

Formula volumes need to increase according to your baby's age and how much breastmilk you are offering. If you are on a feeding plan for weight gain, then the information here won't be as relevant for you. Please talk to your care provider if you have worries or questions about formula amounts.

According to the NHS in the UK:

Newborn babies need quite small amounts of formula to start with. By the end of their first week, most will need around 150 to 200 ml per kilo of their weight a day until they're 6 months old. This amount will vary from baby to baby.

However, the First Steps Nutrition Trust (FSNT) has what I think is a clearer guide, where they break down the volumes suggested according to age. The following is reproduced with their kind permission:

Up to 2 Weeks of Age

7-8 feeds per day of 60-70 ml per feed (around 2 – 2.5 us fl oz)

A total of about 420-560 ml per day (approx. 14 – 18.5 us fl oz)

Breastfed babies are likely to feed much more frequently, and that is perfectly normal.

2 to 8 Weeks

6-7 feeds per day, 75-105 ml per feed (approx 2.5 – 3.5 us fl oz)

Total of 450-735 ml per day (aprox 15 – 25 us fl oz)

2 to 3 Months (9 to 14 Weeks)

5-6 feeds per day 105-180 ml per feed (approx. 3.5 – 6 us fl oz)

525-1,080 ml per day (around 18 – 36.5 us fl oz)

3 to 5 Months (15 to 25 Weeks)

5 feeds per day 180-210 ml per feed (6 – 7.1 fl oz)

900-1,050 ml per day (30.4 – 35.5 fl oz)

About 6 Months (26 Weeks)

4 feeds per day 210-240 ml per feed (7.1 – 8.11 fl oz)

840-960 ml per day (28.5 – 32.4 fl oz)

7 to 9 Months

Infant formula could be offered at breakfast (150 ml), lunch (150 ml), tea (150 ml), and before bed (150 ml). (150 ml is around 5fl oz)

About 600 ml per day (about 20 fl oz)

10 to 12 Months

Infant formula could be offered at breakfast (100 ml), tea (100 ml), and before bed (200 ml). (100 ml is 3.38 fl oz and 200 ml is 6.7 fl oz)

About 400 ml per day (13.5 fl oz)

1 to 2 Years

Full-fat cows' milk could be offered at snack times twice a day (100 ml x 2) and as a drink before bed (200 ml).

About 350-400 ml per day of full-fat cows' milk or other suitable animal milk or milk alternative. Seek advice if using plant-based milk alternatives as these are lower in energy than full-fat animal milk.

(First Steps Nutrition Trust, 2020, 17)

So, how much formula or expressed milk does your combi-fed baby need?

Of course, we can't take any volumes as gospel. Remember that babies need different amounts of formula depending on how much they are breastfeeding, how hungry they are, whether they are thirsty, their age, if they're in a growth spurt, and their weight.

Typically, after the first month of life, a baby will take between 750 and 900 ml of breastmilk a day. To work out how much milk is

needed per feed, we divide the total by the number of feeds baby has. For example: 900 ml/10 feeds = 90ml per feed.

However, this is only a guide. Your baby may take less, or more!

Pacing bottle-feeds can be a useful tool to avoid baby overfeeding when you are mixed feeding. Rather than relying on an amount of milk decided by a general rule, paced feeds given in response to hunger cues allow your baby to tell you whether they are full or not. There are some great online videos easily accessible which demonstrate paced bottle feeding.

Preparation

Formula comes in two forms. Either it is powdered, and you mix it with water for each feed, or it comes ready to feed (RTF) in a bottle or carton. There is a significant difference in price between powdered formula and RTF, and there is now some thinking that RTF may be preferred for newborns or babies with underlying health problems because it's less likely to be contaminated. However, it is a lot less kind to the environment. Some people choose to use it when travelling or when water for powdered formula isn't safe or available.

Preparing powdered formula:

1. Make sure that all equipment is clean and sterile.

    ◊ Sterilising fluid is diluted in water, then bottles, etc., are kept in a large container filled with the solution. The lid should be kept on, and the solution should be changed every day. The bottles don't need to be dried before using them.

    ◊ Pan sterilising is where you boil the bottles and equipment in a pan of water. Once you take the items out, they will need to be used as soon as possible if you want them to stay sterile.

    ◊ Many bottles allow you to sterilise them in the microwave. Follow the manufacturer's instructions.

⬦ Steam sterilisers are either electric or go in the microwave. They typically ask you to keep the bottles inside the device until you want to use each one to maintain hygiene levels that are as high as possible.

⬦ The reason we sterilise equipment is because formula can breed bacteria quicker than breastmilk. Powdered formula, in particular, may carry bacteria that could be harmful to the baby. Sterilising equipment ensures any residue from the formula is thoroughly removed.

2. Boil a full kettle and allow the water to cool to around 70o C (this takes about 10 minutes).

⬦ Many people think we boil the water to kill bacteria in it, but actually, it's to kill anything unwanted in the formula. 70°C is a bit of a compromise since it will kill most of the bad bacteria while keeping most of the nutrients safe. Mixing boiling water with the powder risks destroying some of the nutritional properties in the formula, and your baby needs all of these properties.

3. Wash your hands and make sure anything touching the bottle is freshly cleaned.

4. Fill the bottle with the required amount of water, and then add the instructed number of scoops of powder.

5. Mix the formula by shaking the bottle hard.

6. You can now cool the bottle quickly under a running tap or by standing it in a jug of cold water.

7. Check the temperature by allowing a drop of milk to fall onto your inner wrist. It should be about body temperature, meaning that if you close your eyes while dripping the milk onto your wrist, you won't feel it. It can be a little warmer, or it can be colder – the main thing to avoid is the milk being so hot it burns the baby's mouth.

8. The risk of burns is why we don't heat formula in the microwave. Parts of the formula can get hotter than others, making "hot spots," which may go unnoticed until the baby gets a mouthful a little way into the feed.

IMPORTANT

◊ **Always use a fresh, clean bottle for every feed.**

◊ **Follow the preparation instructions on the tin carefully.**

◊ **Never save unused milk for the next feed.**

A Word on Formula Preparation Machines

These machines work by delivering a small shot of hot water into the bottle before mixing it with cooler water, making the bottle ready to feed to the baby much faster. However, they are not proven safe and are categorically not recommended by various health agencies. They fear that the hotshot is too small and will cool instantly as it comes into contact with the powder, therefore not killing enough bacteria to be safe. Mould is often found in the machines as well, so they do need to be cleaned, and the parts are replaced regularly. The machines are also incredibly expensive for what they are.

Alternatives

It seems dismissive not to acknowledge that the formula preparation machines are popular with families because they save so much time. Goodness knows you want feeds to be offered as fast as possible at 2 am or when the baby is screaming.

An alternative to such a machine could be to feed your baby RTF milks at these times where a bottle is needed immediately. Or, you might want to take a thermos of hot water to bed with you and simply add the already hot water to the milk once the baby wakes. This will save you getting out of bed to put the kettle on, and you could cool the milk in a jug of cold water waiting on the side.

> **Formula preparation machines are not generally recommended due to safety concerns. It is safer for formula to be made as and when it is needed with fresh water from the kettle.**

Storage

UK guidance from the NHS states that formula should be prepared and fed right away to your baby. It used to be that parents were told to make up the entire days' worth of feed and leave it in the fridge, but we now know this increases the risk of the baby becoming unwell if it's done as standard because bacteria can begin to multiply.

The one time when the NHS does suggest making milk up in advance and storing in the fridge is when you will be taking the baby to daycare who won't mix the milk for you and you don't have access to/can't afford ready to feed formula.

The formula must always be made the hot water (70°C is the standard recommendation on formula preparation instructions) so that you kill any bacteria in the powder. If you need to make it in advance, as described above, then it should be cooled as quickly as possible in a bowl of cold water and then stored in the fridge until it is needed. It can then be reheated and fed to the baby. Once reheated, though, it must be used right away and not used after an hour. Milked stored in the fridge as described above should be used as soon as possible, and certainly within 24 hours.

Risks

 Please do skip this section if it's an upsetting topic for you.

After some debate, I decided to include this part of the book. I strongly believe in informed choice, and an essential part of informed choice is having access to everything you possibly can. even where this information might be uncomfortable to read. What follows is a list of known risks related to formula-feeding. I invite you to read up on the cited studies as well for more in-depth reading.

⬥ Sudden Infant Death Syndrome

SIDS is the term that puts fear into all parents. Luckily, it's rare these days because we are so much more aware of safe sleep practices. Breastfeeding for at least two months appears to reduce the risk of SIDS further. A breastfed baby is two times less likely to die from SIDS than a formula-fed baby. The Lullaby Trust has lots of information about safe sleep and reducing the risk of SIDS.

⬥ Allergy

It has been suggested that giving a baby formula in the first days of life may increase the chance of them developing an allergy (Host & Halken, 2014).

One of the amazing things that colostrum does is coat the intestines. Formula doesn't have these antibodies, and the milk can go right through the gaps in the intestinal wall. You might see symptoms like colic or fussiness, vomiting, eczema, a sniffly nose, wheezing, or coughing if your baby has an allergy.

⬥ Breastfeeding Protects from Obesity

The WHO states that breastfeeding protects against obesity and that the chances of obesity decrease the more a baby is breastfed.

⬦ Asthma

Asthma is the most common chronic health problem in childhood, with 14% of school-age children suffering from the condition (Pearce et al., 2007). Children who receive breastmilk seem to be less likely to develop asthma. It also appears that breastfeeding is dose-related. This means that the more the baby is breastfed, the less likely it appears to be that they will develop asthma.

Many studies have been carried out, with some finding no link and a few even discussing an increase in risk with breastfeeding. A systematic review in 2014 looked at over 100 of these studies and concluded that "more vs less breastfeeding" was linked to a 22% decrease in the risk of the child developing asthma (Dogaru et al., 2014).

⬦ Gastroenteritis

Because the living parts of breastmilk go directly into the gut, they are often particularly good at killing nasty bugs that might grow there. This means that we have a clear link between the daily amount of breastfeeding and a reduction in the likelihood of a baby being admitted to hospital with diarrhoea. According to a 2006 study, partial breastfeeding reduces the risk by 25%, and exclusive breastfeeding reduces it by 53% (Quigley et al., 2006).

⬦ Ear Infections

Rather than comparing formula to human milk, the question here relates to bottle-feeding, regardless of what is in the bottle. A 2016 study found that a "longer duration" of bottle-feeding expressed milk saw an increased chance of the baby developing an ear infection compared to their peers who were only feeding at the breast (Boone et al., 2016).

I think a great take-home point for all about the health risks discussed in this section is that the protective element of breastmilk is still there with any breastfeeding and becomes more powerful the more breastmilk is given. The issue of breastmilk or formula feeding isn't as black and white as we are sometimes led to believe. It certainly seems that it's 100% worth continuing to offer as much breastmilk as you are able to or desire while using formula milk.

◊ Financial Burden

While many in the West are fortunate to have enough money to buy infant formula, we really should address the costs that do come along with it. Formula is a market that provides significant profits for those who manufacture it.

The WHO Code of Marketing of Breastmilk Substitutes (the Code) was written in 1981 and has been regularly updated since. It aims to prevent the inappropriate promotion of breastmilk substitutes and protect families, however, they choose to feed their infants. Sadly, the UK, like many other countries, only has a few aspects of the Code in law, and therefore marketing of products and brands to families continues.

The cost of infant milks in the UK is highly variable, and you can see current prices at www.infantmilkinfo.org/costs/.

However, with a tin of formula (which will last about a week if you're exclusively formula-feeding) in the UK costing £10 and up, in addition to the bottles, you will need sterilising fluid, new teats, extra water for cleaning, not to mention the cost of extra use on your kettle, we can quickly find that we are spending a lot of money.

Of course, just like everything else in this section, the effects are dose-related. The more formula you use, the greater the expense. The more you can breastfeed or access donor milk, the more money you can save. Those of us involved in infant feeding support are often frustrated at how challenging accessing help to breastfeed can be, particularly when we know that making this support universally accessible to everyone who needs it would positively impact many areas of family life, including finances.

> The importance of breastmilk is not wiped out by mixed feeding.

◊ **Feelings of Guilt, Failure, or Shame**

———————————— 〝 ————————————

"The only downside to mixed feeding was having to buy lots of bottles and spend lots of money."

~ Survey response

I couldn't write this book and not discuss such an important yet often overlooked topic. Infant feeding is so emotionally loaded that even if you have happily made the choice to use formula, you might be experiencing some difficult or uncomfortable feelings. These feelings are likely to be a lot more pronounced if you have ended up supplementing with formula or donor milk when you want to exclusively breastfeed.

The mums I speak to often describe feeling that they have been starving their baby, that they have failed them, and that Mum herself is a failure – her body has let her down again in a society where she already takes up too much space. Below are some quotes from mums who combination-fed when they wanted to exclusively breastfeed:

> Apart from the lack of support, the cost of formula, the hassle of sterilising bottles, and the disappointment of not being able to EBF, I felt a bit of a failure.

> Felt I had no choice, began to hate that he wasn't getting just my milk. I understand that initially, it helped his blood sugars (10lb1 and blood sugars dropped day 2 – no diabetes

involved), and I am grateful but knowing what I know now, we could have got away from top-ups sooner.

I felt sad that I was led to believe I wasn't making enough milk for my baby. It fed into body image and body confidence issues about small breasts (resulting in years of insecurity, depression, relationship problems, and ultimately surgery). I was sad I hadn't done the natural thing and fed my baby myself.

These quotes tell us quite a story regarding feelings of failure, grief, and guilt. This is a topic that Professor Amy Brown discusses in great detail in her book, *Why Breastfeeding Grief and Trauma Matter* (Brown, 2019).

The problem is not that you have failed as a mother or parent. You are doing the best thing for your baby by ensuring they are fed and growing well while also providing the all-important antibodies and immunological factors in breastmilk. The problem is that the society you live in has failed you and your baby. The truly sad thing about this is people just don't understand that the support they received around breastfeeding could have been a lot better in many cases.

Highly skilled, specialised lactation support is not standard in the UK, and it is certainly not guaranteed in an NHS-run hospital or Health Trust. But no one tells you what an IBCLC is, or even who the highest trained and most experienced person is locally to you. You are left assuming that what you had was good enough.

I would go so far as to say that if you ended up stopping or seriously reducing breastfeeding against your wishes, then you did *not* receive highly skilled, good support. The caveat I would add to that statement is you were also well supported if you were helped to understand why breastfeeding exclusively wasn't going to be an option for you. You were well supported in your grief and were talked through your alternative options (including at breast supplementing and donor milk).

I do not see combination-feeding as a failure. I see it as a great way of ensuring the baby gets the immunological factors in breastmilk along with all the other advantages from breastfeeding: comfort, pain relief, and safety. In addition, you, as a parent, have taken a decision regarding someone's health or wellbeing to also provide some nutrition in the form of a perfectly acceptable food source. Until we do live in a world where mothers' desires to breastfeed exclusively are taken seriously, combination-feeding is a fantastic compromise, in my opinion.

Dealing with Guilt or Grief

The themes of grief and guilt run through nearly every single consultation I have with a parent, even when I can happily report to the mum that everything is happening perfectly. It seems we are designed to worry, to second guess ourselves, and to fear that we are doing something awfully wrong with our babies and children. I think the first step in dealing with your feelings is to understand that nearly all of us parents are feeling anxious about something to do with our little ones.

I forever worry that my youngest is going to end up as a criminal mastermind (he is 4, by the way). I'm totally allowed to worry about that, and it's also helpful for me to step back and understand that the criminal mastermind scenario is just a story my brain is telling me to try to keep said 4-year-old safe. It helps to distance myself.

Mindfulness can also be helpful. The wonderful Anna Le Grange, who is a mindfulness coach as well as an IBCLC with personal experience of combination-feeding, has kindly given me this script to share with you as well as a link to download and listen to her meditation.

Find somewhere comfortable to be where you can spend 10 quiet minutes to yourself. You can be seated or lying down, whatever feels best for you right now. You might want to use extra cushions or pillows to help you relax more deeply. Maybe behind your head or the back of your knees.

If you feel able to, gently close your eyes and start to take your focus inwards. Taken a few nice, slow, deep breaths now and feel them start to settle down. Become aware of how your body changes as you breathe in and then out, abdomen and ribs both moving with the breath.

And noticing too, how the air feels as it enters and then leaves again, feeling it at the edge or insides of your nostrils and then as it comes down your nasal cavity and back of your throat before heading down into your lungs.

Breathing naturally, however, your body wants to do it, in and out.

And as you continue, feeling the ground beneath you, feeling your weight on the ground.

In and out.

Sending your focus down to your feet now. Focussing on them on your next in-breath and then as you breathe out, feeling your feet relax fully.

Sending your focus to your legs now. Focussing on them on your next in-breath and then as you breathe out, feeling your legs relax fully.

Sending your focus down to your hips and belly now. Focussing on them on your next in-breath and then as you breathe out, feeling your hips and belly relax fully.

Taking your focus down to your chest now. Focussing on it on your next in-breath, and then as you breathe out, feeling your chest relax fully.

Taking your focus to your back now. Focussing on it on your next in-breath, and then as you breathe out, feeling your back relax fully.

Taking your focus to your arms and hands now. Focussing on them on your next in-breath and then as you breathe out, feeling your arms and hands relax fully.

Taking your focus to your neck and shoulders. Focussing on them on your next in-breath, and then as you breathe out, feeling your neck and shoulders relax fully.

And finally taking your focus to your face. Focusing on it during your next in-breath and then as you breathe out, feeling your face relax.

Your whole body is now feeling calm and relaxed. Breathing steady, and as you sit or lay here silently and peacefully, your deeper mind is more open to positive thoughts or affirmations. This is the perfect time to think positively about all that you are doing.

I'm going to repeat some positive phrases to you now. Some will resonate with you, and some may not. That's ok. Just repeat the phrases silently to yourself. All the time remembering to breathe.

I am the best parent for my baby.

I feel calm and relaxed as I feed my baby.

This breastfeeding journey is between my baby and me.

I trust my body and my baby.

I ask for help when I need it.

I trust my instincts.

I nourish myself so that I can nourish my baby.

I control what I can and let go of the rest.

I take it one day at a time.

I am grateful for what my body is able to do.

My baby and I have a unique bond that is not shared by anyone else.

I have a deep connection with my baby that is not shared with anyone else in the world.

Taking a deep breath now. Right into the bottom of your lungs. And then letting it go.

And again, deep breath in and release.

Feeling a sense of positivity and wellbeing surrounding you and your whole body.

Thanking your body and your mind for this moment of self-care.

Now slowly becoming aware of your surroundings again. Noticing any external noises.

Wiggling your fingers and your toes if you feel ready.

Staying in bed for a nap or the night's sleep if you wish.

If you're going to get up now, just slowly moving around more and opening your eyes if you feel ready.

Find something to focus on in the room. Remind yourself where you are."

Anna Le Grange IBCLC

The Mindful Breastfeeding School

The download of this relaxation can be found here: *https://www.themindfulbreastfeedingschool.com/freebies*

Grief and Guilt

We cannot talk about combination-feeding without acknowledging that many parents will experience feelings of grief and/or guilt regarding the use of formula. This seems to be the case even where combination-feeding was a choice made free from pressure. Dr Amy Brown has written a book on this topic called *Why Breastfeeding Grief and Trauma Matter.* It's a great place to start to look more deeply at the feelings you might be dealing with.

Grief around breastfeeding is something I see in my work on a daily basis and seems to be a logical consequence of telling mothers how important breastfeeding is and then not providing them with the support and information they need to actually meet their goals. One thing I am confident about, having spent 18 years working with families of young children, is that children love their parents and vice versa. The way we feed our babies is one part of parenting, and we don't need to breastfeed exclusively to ensure close attachment and well-rounded children.

I am still, after all this time, struck by the eye contact between the mum and baby during feeding: whether that's with a bottle or breast. The pair gaze at each other deeply; the mum smiling, cooing, and making exaggerated facial expressions designed subconsciously to teach communication skills and strengthen the attachment between the dyad. You're doing a good job, Mama. You are.

If your feelings of sadness, grief, or guilt are strong, or they aren't going away with time, then you might find talking things through with a professional helpful. This could be through formal counselling or even from a breastfeeding counsellor on one of the many national helplines available in the UK and around the rest of the world.

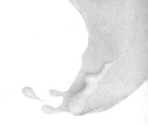

CHAPTER 4

Human Milk and Informal Milk Sharing

You may not be aware of informal milk sharing as an option for feeding your baby. This is where you receive donated milk from other breastfeeding mothers, and you give this to your baby instead of formula. Often, the initial reaction from parents when informal milk sharing is first suggested is disgust, but if we take a moment to unpick this, it may feel less weird.

Formula is made from cows' milk, which is widely accepted as normal in our culture, even though, as a species, we probably aren't designed to drink the milk from another mammal. Certainly, in cultures where cows' milk is not widely used for human consumption, people tend to be lactose intolerant as adults. Human milk is just milk made for human babies to consume. Human milk is designed for human babies, while cows' milk is designed for calves.

Even though human milk is made for human babies, it is still important that you weigh up the option of milk sharing thoroughly before you decide. There are some potential risks to milk sharing. Let's explore the things to be aware of below:

Pros

◊ Donor milk is free.

◊ Your baby continues to be exclusively breastfed, which comes with improved health outcomes.

◊ It may be easier to source allergen-free breastmilk than a prescription formula.

◊ You will be contributing to the normalisation of human milk.

◊ It is more environmentally friendly.

Things to Be Aware of

◊ You have to trust that the donor has good hygiene standards regarding expressing and storing her milk.

◊ You need to trust her to disclose any medications or dietary preferences honestly.

◊ It's been known for women to dilute their milk with formula, cows' milk, or water to make it go further. This is more likely to be a problem where human milk is being sold rather than donated.

◊ You may well be meeting a stranger who isn't who they say they are.

◊ In theory, the donor may have a disease incompatible with breast-feeding, such as Hepatitis or unmanaged HIV. However, this is unlikely as she wouldn't be breastfeeding her own baby in this instance.

◊ Sometimes babies won't drink milk that has been frozen and defrosted.

◊ Generally speaking, people who are donating their milk are genuine mums who are keen to support other women to give their babies breastmilk. Particularly where donated milk is involved, the risks seem to be incredibly low, with few problems reported from donor or recipient. Often, you're doing the donor a favour by helping her to free up freezer space without her having to throw away the milk she worked hard to express.

History of Donor Milk

As mentioned previously, before we had a safe alternative to breast-milk, donor milk was often provided in the form of a wet nurse. We have evidence dating back to 2000 BC of wet nurses being used. The Babylonians even had a strict set of rules for these women to adhere to, which provide us with the first known evidence of such a code of conduct (Moro, 2018).

Of course, the history of wet nursing is riddled with serious human rights problems. Throughout history impoverished and enslaved women have been used to feed the babies of those with more power. It is important that we are open about this history and that any discussion involving using other people's milk includes acknowledgement of this deeply problematic past. For more on the topic of slavery and wet nursing a google search will pull up dozens of articles from black and brown people, and they are far more qualified than anyone to discuss this.

Theodor Escherich, of the University of Vienna, carried out studies between 1902 and 1911 on the different sorts of milk babies were fed. He found that breastfed babies had different gut bacteria to babies fed on other milks. In 1909, he opened the first-ever milk bank, and the following year, the first American milk bank opened at the Boston Floating Hospital (Haiden, Ekhard, & Ziegler, 2016).

Informal milk sharing seems to be today's equivalent of wet nursing (although the practice of feeding someone else's baby is still in action, it tends to be more private in our culture and rarely spoken about openly). While there are now many milk banks all over the world, and mothers frequently donate to their local one, the milk collected is usually saved for the most vulnerable, premature, or sick babies where breastmilk is not available to them.

Mums who find themselves with an unneeded freezer stash of their own pumped milk won't meet the strict criteria of pre-screening for donating this milk formally. So they may turn to the informal milk sharing websites and groups on the web to donate their milk to others in need.

Matthias's Story

This story, kindly shared by Matthias, beautifully illustrates how and why donor milk can be used instead of, or as well as, formula.

> Isabella was born in August 2019, thanks to the help of an altruistic surrogate. From the moment she was born, she was cared for by her two fathers.

Thanks to more than 50 generous women, we have been able to almost exclusively give Isabella donated human breastmilk during the first six months of her life. Milk sharing is recommended by The World Health Organization and UNICEF if a mother's own milk is not available. The next best thing is the milk of another woman, according to the WHO.

When we were pregnant and first looking into given donor breastmilk, we knew very little about milk sharing. However, it seems that there is a very big community out there on different kinds of platforms. Thanks to various sites and social media, we found women who had an oversupply of breastmilk and who would happily pump for our little munchkin. From some women, we have collected more than 15 litres over the past months. From some women, we have collected half a litre. For each drop of milk, we have been grateful.

Once Isabella had turned 6 months, we switched to formula. This was because we believe the (unfortunately) little available donor milk should go to younger babies in need. To the women out there who have an oversupply: please consider donating your milk. This liquid gold could make a difference to the start of a young baby. And to the parents in need, please do have a look into milk sharing as breast is best!

All About Breastmilk: How It Works

There is no denying that breastmilk is pretty cool. It is the only food in the world that adapts to the needs of the individual drinking it. If the weather is hot, breastmilk becomes more watery to support hydration. If it's cold out, the milk becomes higher in fat to support the extra calorie needs for warmth. If the mother has contact with a virus, the antibodies to that virus find their way into her milk and then into her baby. This is why breastfeeding reduces the risk of baby catching gastroenteritis, and if they do catch it, they seem to recover faster than exclusively formula-fed babies.

Breastmilk is made on a demand-and-supply basis (as opposed to the supply-and-demand basis often discussed). Essentially, if the milk is not demanded, it won't carry on being supplied. Much like if a shop realises its sales of eggs has dropped off, it will stop stocking them.

This demand and supply works so well thanks to a whey protein in human milk called Feedback Inhibitor of Lactation, or FIL for short. The job of FIL is to slow down milk production if milk isn't being used, so the breast doesn't become dangerously full. So, the more milk in the breast, the more FIL is also present, telling the body to apply the milk-making brakes. Essentially, if you don't remove milk, you won't make more milk.

This is relevant for combination-feeding because if you want to keep a degree of breastfeeding going long term, it's important that you, well, breastfeed. The awesome thing about breastmilk is that your body will adapt to a change in demand. Think about a mother breastfeeding her 2-year-old: the toddler is at nursery five days a week and doesn't breastfeed while away from Mum. Yet, they still enjoy a breastfeeding relationship in the evenings, at night, and on the weekends. Mum's body has adjusted to the change in demand, and now makes just the right amount of milk for her little one's needs.

Prolactin is also important for us to understand and discuss here. Prolactin is the hormone that tells your breasts to make milk. It can only do this when it's at a high enough level. Breastfeeding increases levels of prolactin each time you put the baby to the breast. Those levels reach their peak 45 minutes later and then fall steadily until they return to baseline.

In order to keep making milk, we need to avoid those levels plummeting to baseline. While feeding at least eight times a day is recommended for exclusive breastfeeding, you can breastfeed less and keep prolactin high enough to keep making milk. It has been suggested that prolactin drops back to baseline after about six hours of no stimulation. Never going longer than 6 hours between feeds, (and aiming to feed MORE often) should keep enough of a milk supply that you don't run into problems. That's 4-6 feeds per 24 hours. Having said this, if you suddenly start going a long time between feeds and your breasts become full, milk production may slow down more than you want it to.

Having said this, everyone is different. We do need to exercise a degree of caution with combination feeding and I would strongly recommend taking things slowly so that if you notice that supply is dropping or baby is becoming fussy at the breast it will be easier to adjust things back into the favour of breastfeeding. In addition to this some babies will become tricky to feed at the breast if lots of bottles are being given so be sure to watch for signs of increased or new challenges, try to use a cup if possible, and if bottle feeding is the way forward for them please do remember paced feeding.

The brilliant thing about breastmilk is, if you feel that your supply is dropping, you can begin to breastfeed or pump more often to raise prolactin and reduce FIL, and this will tell your body to make more milk within a few days. This is also why you can also return to full breastfeeding if you are someone combi-feeding through necessity rather than a choice, or if circumstances change, and it makes sense to breastfeed more than formula-feed (for example, during the sort of formula shortage we saw in the COVID-19 panic buying).

It will take several days for you to notice your milk supply beginning to increase. Still, as long as you are consistent with feeding more frequently, and you don't have an underlying issue preventing full milk supply, then your milk is likely to increase in volume according to demand.

> It's a good idea, where possible, to introduce formula or donor milk slowly, one feed every 3 to 5 days, so your body can adjust to the change in demand at the right pace.

Causes of Low Supply

Ineffective Milk Removal

This is the most common reason for low milk supply, and it can often be overcome with the right sort of help where a return to exclusive breastfeeding is desired. When the baby isn't able to remove milk often and well, the body gets a message that it needs to make less. A deep latch is essential to good milk removal as it helps the baby to strip the milk away from the milk ducts in an effective way that doesn't cause pain for Mum or tiredness and/or frustration for the baby.

I know I mention this a lot, but that's because it is the most important part of breastfeeding. If your baby has a shallow latch, *seek support* from someone well trained in breastfeeding care and remember that such a person may not be accessible as part of your standard care.

Possible Signs of Ineffective Milk Removal

- ⬦ The baby's chin is not touching the breast during feeds.
- ⬦ You cannot hear regular swallowing.
- ⬦ The baby is gaining weight slowly.
- ⬦ The baby frequently pulls off the breast and cries.
- ⬦ The baby frequently falls asleep within minutes of latching.
- ⬦ Less than two dirty nappies per day in the first six weeks of life.
- ⬦ Lack of heavy wet nappies with light-coloured urine inside them.
- ⬦ The baby slips off the breast after latching well.
- ⬦ The baby clicks repeatedly while feeding.
- ⬦ Milk pours out of the side of the mouth or nose.
- ⬦ Nipples are blanched, pinched, or slanted after feeds.
- ⬦ Nipples are cracked, blistered, or bleeding.
- ⬦ You have frequent engorgement, blocked ducts, or mastitis.
- ⬦ It feels as though the baby is clamping or chomping on your nipple.

Many of these things on their own, or in a different context, may tell us something else. For example, pulling off and crying shortly into a feed may also be a sign of oversupply, and some babies are good feeders despite what looks like a shallow latch. Therefore, good support is important to help you work out what the issue is and also what is causing the ineffective milk removal. Is it "just" positioning and attachment? Is it a tongue-tie? A weak or disorganised suck? Does the baby have some soreness or tension from birth?

Infrequent Milk Removal

As above, if the breast isn't stimulated often, then it will begin to make less milk to adjust to the decreased need. Infrequent milk removal can be due to the baby being sleepy and not feeding as often as they should, or it could be because the family are trying to feed the baby according to a routine or are using a dummy a lot of the time. Remember that the guidance now is to feed babies responsively: if they are acting hungry, they need feeding. We don't need to stretch them to a certain length of time.

Retained Placenta

Full milk production is kickstarted by the delivery of the placenta. This is due to the sharp shift in different hormones. It only takes a small piece of the placenta to be retained for those hormones to not do their shifting. In this case, the mum may find that despite the days ticking by, her milk isn't coming in. It can be reassuring to know that once the placenta is fully removed, milk supply often increases.

Hypothyroidism

Speller and Brodribb (2012) state that there is a link between hypothyroidism and low milk supply.

Symptoms of hypothyroidism include:

- ◊ Tiredness
- ◊ Low blood pressure
- ◊ Obesity
- ◊ Dry skin
- ◊ Feeling the cold

If hypothyroidism is possible, then please see your doctor. Once the correct medication is prescribed and begins to work, milk volume usually increases.

Polycystic Ovary Syndrome

Polycystic Ovary Syndrome (PCOS) affects about 5% to 10% of women. It can be caused by both genetic and environmental factors. PCOS is a big cause of infertility and has many symptoms and associated problems, including:

- Increased risk of type 2 diabetes
- Excessive hair
- Irregular periods
- Light periods
- No periods
- Obesity

PCOS has an unpredictable effect on breastfeeding. Some people experience no problems at all, while others struggle with low supply—a fairly good indicator of whether you will experience problems or not are breast changes during pregnancy. Breast changes are associated with fewer problems (Vanky et al., 2012).

Metformin is a medication used to help manage PCOS, and some women say they have found that taking this increases breast milk production.

Hypoplasia or IGT

Hypoplasia of the breast, or insufficient glandular tissue (IGT), are the terms we may use when talking about breasts that have less tissue than is needed to make a full milk supply. There is a broad spectrum of IGT, from no milk being produced to a nearly full supply and every possible scenario in between. The causes of IGT range from simple anatomy, poor development in adolescence due to malnutrition (for example, from an eating disorder), and Polycystic Ovary Syndrome. Interestingly, more breast tissue is often laid down in subsequent pregnancies, meaning that the more babies a mum has, the more likely it is that she can breastfeed.

Breast Surgery (Or Any Surgery Involving the Intercostal Nerves)

Breast reduction surgery can either cause big problems or no problems at all. It depends on the type of procedure carried out and how long ago it occurred.

Breast Augmentation Surgery

Firstly, let's consider breast implants or breast augmentation. Many mothers who have breast implants go on to breastfeed exclusively, with one study saying up to 80% of the mums they worked with produced a full milk supply. Frustratingly, this study was carried out by breast surgeons who may have a vested interest in women thinking surgery won't affect their ability to breastfeed (Jewell et al., 2019).

Although many women can breastfeed just fine following augmentation, the reason for the surgery can tell us more. Surgery because breasts were an unusual shape or lacked glandular tissue will possibly be masking a physiological reason for long-term low supply.

We also need to bear in mind the likelihood of scarring or breast tissue damage because of the surgery carried out. Broadly, it is considered that implants behind the breast (inframammary implants) are less likely to have a negative impact on breastfeeding because usually, the tissue and nerves are left intact. Axillary enlargement (under the armpit) also tends to leave the nerves and tissue untouched. The Periareola method is where an incision is made around the areola. This is much more likely to result in nerve damage, and one report cites that women with this type of incision are more likely to struggle with breastfeeding (Neifert et al., 1990).

Another issue to consider here is maternal confidence. Sometimes the reasons women seek breast implants are related to a dislike of their body, which may also come with feelings of mistrust. If you don't trust your breasts to do their job, perhaps you will be more likely to think a problem can't be overcome.

Regardless of possible issues, the best chance of successful exclusive breastfeeding following breast augmentation will be with good, early support regarding milk removal.

Breast Reduction Surgery

As with breast implants, the type of surgery will depend on the likelihood of successful breastfeeding, along with good support to maximise milk removal in the early days.

Liposuction is where fat is removed from the breast. This is the technique least likely to cause problems, although some glandular tissue may be damaged.

The inferior-pedicle technique is sometimes called the anchor technique, as it leaves an anchor-shaped scar around the base of the areola and down the breast tissue. This method of breast reduction is also more likely than others to allow a degree of breastfeeding later, as the nipple is left on a mound (or pedicle) of breast tissue, which aims to protect some of the nerves.

Periareola technique, as with breast augmentation, may lead to glandular and nerve damage.

The free-graft technique is the most likely method to lead to an inability to breastfeed. Here, the nipple and areola are completely removed and reattached, severing nerves entirely. No nerves means no sensation to the nipple, and no sensation to the nipple means the body won't get messages from stimulation to produce milk. It is possible, however, that over time some damage may be healed, leading to some sensation in the nipple.

Remember that this book exists to offer support with combination-feeding by choice and through necessity. Even if you produce no or little milk, you can still have a baby at your breast for comfort and connection.

Certain Medications

Hormonal contraceptives are probably the biggest medicinal cause of low milk supply. Even the progesterone-only pill, which is widely considered safe to take six weeks after birth, comes with thousands of anecdotal reports from mums that supply is damaged when taking it. Decongestants are another cause of reduced milk supply that people don't always know about, with some sources claiming that a single dose can reduce supply by 25%. If things are going okay breastfeeding-wise, but you have noticed a decrease in milk volume since starting some medication, it is a good idea to check that the medication isn't the cause. In most cases, once the drug is stopped, milk supply returns.

In the UK, we have a genuinely outstanding source of free support for medicines while breastfeeding. Pharmacologist, Dr. Wendy Jones, runs a service called The Drugs in Breastmilk Information Service, which can be accessed by email or Facebook messenger if you require tailored support. The service also offers many online factsheets if you want to double-check whether something is safe to take or not. Wendy has written several books on this topic and is widely regarded as an expert by both the medical field and volunteers alike.

Sheehan's Syndrome

This particularly tricky condition can happen after a large amount of blood is lost during a postpartum haemorrhage. It is caused by blood pressure becoming so incredibly low that the blood doesn't get as far as the pituitary gland. This means that the cells in the gland stop working or die, and milk stops being made. This damage, sadly, is permanent, and the mum may make a little milk or none at all depending on the damage done.

Human Milk Feeding

Colostrum

Colostrum is the first milk that you make. It's typically present from about halfway through pregnancy in tiny amounts, and once the baby is born, this milk is the first feed they will usually have. It's rich in antibodies – so much so that it's sometimes called the baby's first immunisation. The other awesome thing about colostrum is that it is a great laxative, meaning that it can help the baby to pass that thick, sticky meconium, which is their first bowel movement. Even if you don't want to breastfeed, colostrum can be collected in late pregnancy and fed to the baby by a syringe to give them a highly concentrated shot of antibodies and laxatives.

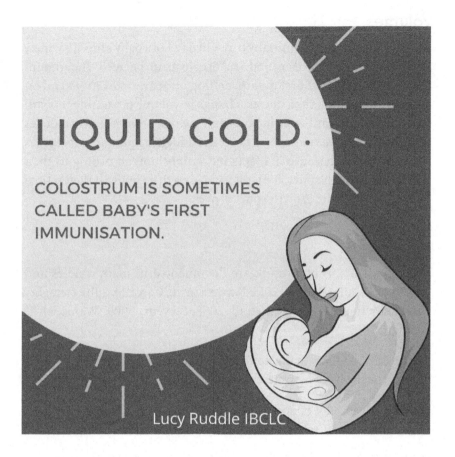

Mature Milk

Over the first week, milk increases in volume, changes colour, and becomes waterier in appearance. Mature milk is what your baby takes once that transition is completed, right up until their last breastfeed. Mature milk changes in composition throughout the course of lactation, adapting to the baby's needs as they grow. One particularly amazing fact about breastmilk is that as your baby weans. It takes less milk over time, some of the immunoglobulins in milk become more concentrated, therefore providing more immunological support for the child as they begin to explore more of the world and come into contact with more germs.

Volumes

Breastmilk volumes are initially tiny. On day 1 of a baby's life, it's widely cited that they only need around 5 ml of colostrum per feed. The amount then increases for the first month, ending up at around 750-900 ml on average. Breastmilk then doesn't change in volume (assuming it is still being removed) until weaning begins, at which point it slowly reduces in quantity. The reason babies don't need higher and higher volumes of breastmilk is because it adapts its composition according to their needs. In a growth spurt, it might increase a little but will then return to baseline after the growth spurt is over.

Ingredients

The ingredients in breastmilk are documented in many studies and books (Aloe, 2015; Bodnar, 2013; Bonyata, n. d.; Garofalo, 2010; Geraghty, 2013; kellymom.com; Owen et al., 2008; Stevens, 2009; Wambach & Riordan, 2016).

Water. Breastmilk is made up from a lot of water (About 88%), which keeps the baby hydrated.

Lactose. Meets a lot of energy needs and may help with the absorption of some minerals like Calcium and Zinc.

Carboxylic acid, Alpha hydroxy acid, and Lactic acid. These are fatty acids, which can provide energy and transport fat-soluble nutrients.

Casein and Whey Protein. Breast milk contains casein and whey proteins. Their levels change as lactation continues. Casein is low in early lactation, then rapidly rises. Whey levels are high in the beginning, then gradually decrease. Casein proteins are slow to digest. By contrast, whey proteins are very quickly and easily digested, providing the baby with continuous nutrition.

Alpha-lactalbumin. This is the most common whey protein in breast milk. It has pain-relieving, anti-microbial and anti-viral properties. When it is exposed to stomach acid, it changes its composition to become HAMLET (Human Alpha-lactalbumin Made Lethal to Tumour) cells. HAMLET cells have been observed to cause the death of cancer cells, and research is ongoing as to their potential use as a treatment for cancer.

Lactoferrin. This has an anti-tumour effect and significantly inhibits the growth of certain cancerous cells. It is an iron-binding protein, which helps babies to absorb iron but also prevents harmful microorganisms from absorbing the iron they need to survive. It inhibits infection by Hepatitis B; Hepatitis C; Adenovirus, which causes the common cold; Respiratory Syncytial Virus (RSV), and many more.

Serum albumin. One of the major components of whey protein, this provides essential amino acids.

Creatine. Creatine is an amino acid that can help recharge energy in muscle cells.

Peptides (see below)

Amino Acids (the building blocks of proteins). Amino acids combine to make proteins and peptides. Of the twenty amino acids, our bodies can only naturally produce eleven, the other nine, the essential amino acids must come from our diet. Amino acids have a wide range of functions, including building muscles, causing chemical reactions in the body, and transporting nutrients around the body.

- ⬦ **Alanine.** Helps the body digest sugars to provide energy for muscles, the brain, and the central nervous system.
- ⬦ **Arginine.** This causes the release of growth hormones that helps build and repair muscles.
- ⬦ **Aspartate.** A non-essential amino acid, it is one of the building blocks of proteins and peptides.
- ⬦ **Glycine.** A non-essential amino acid, one of the building blocks of proteins, it's also a neurotransmitter, meaning it helps transmit chemical signals across the brain.

○ **Cystine.** One of the building blocks of proteins and peptides. It is found in m any of the body's tissues.

○ **Glutamate.** This is one of the most abundant amino acids in the brain and works as a neurotransmitter.

○ **Histidine.** Histidine facilitates the creation and growth of blood cells and helps with tissue repair.

○ **Isoleucine.** Isoleucine helps hormone production, blood sugar regulation, and wound healing.

○ **Leucine.** Leucine helps the growth and repair of muscle and bone. It also initiates the production of protein.

○ **Lysine.** Lysine helps build muscle, maintain bone strength, aids recovery from illness and injury, regulates hormones, antibodies, and enzymes, and may have anti-viral properties.

○ **Methionine.** Methionine aids the absorption of selenium and zinc, and helps remove heavy metals like lead and mercury.

○ **Phenylalanine.** Phenylalanine is necessary for certain brain functions. It also helps the body to use other amino acids, as well as proteins and enzymes.

○ **Proline.** Aids with the functioning of joints and tendons, and could strengthen the heart muscles.

○ **Serine.** A non-essential amino acid, one of the building blocks of proteins and peptides.

○ **Taurine.** This is essential for the development of the brain and nervous system.

○ **Theronine.** Theronine is a component of tooth enamel, collagen, and elastine. Therefore, it is essential for healthy skin and teeth.

○ **Tryptophan.**Tryptophan is necessary for proper growth in infants and can help the production of serotonin and melatonin.

○ **Tyrosine.** A non-essential amino acid, this forms the building blocks of proteins and peptides.

⬦ **Valine.** Valine helps muscle coordination.

⬦ **Carnitine.** This helps the body convert fats into energy.

Nucleotides (chemical compounds that are the structural units of RNA and DNA). Nucleotides are the building blocks of DNA and RNA. They are involved in many metabolic processes, and they can also form other structures that activate or inhibit certain processes within the body's cells. For example, many nucleotides are coenzymes, which can help speed up chemical reactions in the body. They play a role in developing and maturing the gastric tract and help the immune system function. They also provide the baby with a source of nitrogen.

Fats. Fat in breast milk provides roughly 50% of the baby's calorie intake. Besides storing energy, fats have a number of other functions, including cell messaging and hormone production. Fat is the most variable component in human milk. The fat content in milk varies depending on what stage of lactation the mother is at, what time of day it is, and from mother to mother. For example, the milk of a mother with a preterm baby contains approximately 30% more fat than the mother of a term baby. The total fat content of breast milk ranges from 22 to 62g/L.

Triglycerides. These are important for the development of the eyes, central nervous system, and the brain and are associated with higher cognitive ability in children. AHA also reduces pain and inflammation. DHA and AHA make up 20% of the fatty acid content of the brain.

⬦ **Linoleic Acid.** An essential fatty acid, which is thought to reduce the risk of heart disease.

⬦ **Alpha-Linolenic Acid (ALA).** An essential fatty acid, which may reduce the risk of heart disease and strokes.

⬦ **Eicosapentaenoic Acid (EPA).** An Omega-3 fatty acid, this may reduce the risk of heart disease.

⬦ **Conjugated Linoleic Acid (Rumenic Acid).** An Omega-6 fatty acid, which may reduce the risk of heart disease.

Free Fatty Acids

Monounsaturated Fatty Acids

◊ **Oleic acid, Palmitoleic acid, Heptadecenoic acid.** These
  may reduce the risk of heart disease

◊ Saturated Fatty Acids

◊ **Stearic, Palmitic acid, Lauric acid, and Myristic acid.**
  These are an essential source of energy and help the body
  absorb certain vitamins and minerals.

◊ Phospholipids

◊ **Phosphatidylcholine, Phosphatidylethanolamine,
  Phosphatidylinositol, Lysophosphatidylcholine, and
  Lysophosphatidylethanolamine.** These play important roles
  in the structure of the body's cells and cell membranes.

◊ **Plasmalogens.** These are important components of the
  immune nervous and cardiovascular systems. They help
  speed up nerve messages.

Sphingolipids

◊ **Glucosylceramide, Glycosphingolipids,
  Galactosylceramide, Lactosylceramide,
  Globotriaosylceramide (GB3), and Globoside (GB4).**
  These help to protect the surfaces of cells, especially nerve
  cells. They have an important role in transmitting signals
  from one cell to another.

◊ **Sphingomyelin.** These form part of cell membranes,
  particularly in the myelin sheath, which covers nerve cells; this
  makes it important for sending signals between different cells.

◊ **Gangliosides, GM1, GM2, GM3.** These are critical to
  normal brain development. They help nerves to repair
  themselves and may have a role in the development of the
  immune system.

Sterols. These are important for all human cell membranes and signalling between cells. Vitamin D metabolites are important for healthy bones, teeth, and muscles. Steroid hormones act as chemical messengers and are important in the development and function of the reproductive system. Cholesterol is used to make bile, which is vital for digestion. Others, such as Squalene, are thought to have antioxidant and anti-tumour properties. See the full list of sterols below:

◊	Squalene	◊	7-dehydrocholesterol
◊	Dimethylsterol	◊	Stigma-and campesterol
◊	Methosterol	◊	7-ketocholesterol
◊	Lathosterol	◊	Sitosterol
◊	Desmosterol	◊	β-lathosterol
◊	Triacylglycerol	◊	Vitamin D metabolites
◊	Cholesterol	◊	Steroid hormones

Vitamins and Minerals. Vitamins and minerals perform a variety of roles. Most are essential for growth and development.

◊ **Vitamin A.** Vitamin A is important for supporting the immune system and for vision and healthy skin

◊ **Vitamin B6.** Makes haemoglobin, the substance in red blood cells that carries oxygen through the body.

◊ **Vitamin B8 (Inositol).** A vitamin-like substance that may help regulate certain body functions.

◊ **Vitamin B12.** B12 makes red blood cells and helps the body absorb folic acid.

◊ **Vitamin C.** Vitamin C supports the immune system and helps the body to absorb Iron.

◊ **Vitamin D.** Vitamin D supports the growth of bones and muscles.

◊ **Vitamin E.** Vitamin E supports the immune system and protects the eyes and skin.

- **a-Tocopherol.** This is a type of E vitamin. It is an antioxidant, and along with other E, vitamin substances can protect the body against many degenerative conditions.

- **Vitamin K.** Vitamin K is needed for blood clotting.

- **Thiamine.** Thiamine is used for turning food into energy.

- **Riboflavin.** Riboflavin keeps the eyes and nervous system healthy.

- **Niacin.** A type of B vitamin – helps to metabolise fats and proteins and helps the nervous system to work properly.

- **Folic acid.** A synthetic form of folate that helps to build DNA.

- **Pantothenic acid.** Also known as vitamin B5. It is necessary for converting food into energy.

- **Biotin.** Biotin helps the body break down fats.

- **Calcium.** Aids with bone development

- **Sodium.** Sodium helps to balance the amount of fluid in the body.

- **Potassium.** Potassium keeps the heart working properly and regulates the amount of fluid in the body.

- **Iron.** Iron is essential for the production of haemoglobin, the oxygen-carrying protein found in red blood cells.

- **Zinc.** Zinc aids in the production of new cells and enzymes wound healing and helps the body process carbohydrates, fat, and protein.

- **Chloride.** Alongside sodium, this helps to regulate the amount of fluid in the body, and aids digestion.

- **Phosphorus.** This is a component of bones, teeth, DNA, and RNA. Also, a component of cell membrane structure and of the body's key energy source, which is called ATP. Lots of proteins and sugars in the body are phosphorylated.

- **Magnesium.** Magnesium helps to convert food into energy and plays a role in bone health and repair.

◊ **Copper.** Copper helps the production of red and white blood cells and triggers the release of iron to form haemoglobin- the protein that transports oxygen around the body.

◊ **Manganese.** Manganese helps to produce and activate certain enzymes.

◊ **Iodine.** Iodine helps the production of thyroid hormones, which in turn keep the body's cells and metabolism healthy.

◊ **Selenium.** Selenium prevents damage to muscles and cells and helps the immune system work properly.

◊ **Choline.** Choline is essential for the development of the brain and nervous system.

◊ **Sulpher.** One of the most abundant minerals in the body, generally provided by the essential amino acid methionine.

◊ **Chromium.** Chromium is thought to affect how insulin behaves and how much energy the body can absorb from food.

◊ **Cobalt.** An essential trace element, it is part of vitamin B-12

◊ **Fluorine.** Important for healthy bones and teeth.

◊ **Nickel.** Affects iron absorption and may help to produce red blood cells.

◊ **Molybdenum.** Molybdenum helps produce and activate enzymes that make and repair genetic material.

Growth Factors. Growth factors in breast milk stimulate the development of certain types of tissue, such as intestinal lining.

Stem Cells. These are cells that can divide and renew to repair different organs and systems. They are absorbed by the baby, but their function remains unknown. Stem cells are currently being used in research for a variety of illnesses.

Cytokines

Interleukin-1β (IL-1β) and IL-2, IL-4, IL-6, IL-8, IL-10. These are a group of molecules that help regulate the immune system and promote responses to infections and inflammation. These are thought to play a significant role in the immune protection properties of breast milk. Most cytokines that newborns are deficient in are found in abundance in breast milk. They bind to specific receptors on cells and aid the development and function of the immune system.

Other factors in breast milk include:

- ◊ **Granulocyte-colony stimulating factor (G-CSF).** This helps the body make more white blood cells.

- ◊ **Macrophage-colony stimulating factor (M-CSF).** This plays an important role in making infection-fighting white blood cells more effective.

- ◊ **Platelet-derived growth factors (PDGF).** These help heal wounds, repair blood vessels walls, and help blood vessels to grow.

- ◊ **Vascular endothelial growth factor (VEGF)**

- ◊ **Hepatocyte growth factor -α (HGF-α)**

- ◊ **HGF-β**

- ◊ **Tumor necrosis factor-α.** This triggers cells, like white blood cells, to begin fighting an infection.

- ◊ **Interferon-γ.** This is crucial to the immune system. It activates and stimulates germ-killing cells.

- ◊ **Epithelial growth factor (EGF).** These have an essential role in wound healing.

- ◊ **Transforming growth factor-α (TGF-α).** This stimulates gastrointestinal growth and repair.

- ◊ **TGF β1 and TGF-β2.** These growth factors promote the development of the gastric tract. They allow the immune system to tolerate exposure to nutrients and healthy bacteria in the gut. They also promote repair of damaged cells in the intestine. This helps to protect the baby from NEC.

◊ **Insulin-like growth factor-I (IGF-I) (also known as somatomedin C) and Insulin-like growth factor- II.** This is thought to promote infant growth.

◊ **Nerve growth factor (NGF).** This plays a key role in neuron development.

◊ **Erythropoietin.** This stimulates stem cells to produce red blood cells.

Peptides (Combinations of Amino Acids). Peptides are like proteins, as they are made up of amino acids, but they're smaller. Research suggests that peptides may be able to kill microbes, reduce inflammation, and improve immune function.

◊ **HMGF I (Human growth factor), HMGF II, HMGF III.** These are messengers on certain cell receptors that stimulate cells to divide and multiply. Epidermal Growth Factor (EMF) is especially important for the development of the digestive tract and protecting babies against NEC (necrotizing enterocolitis).

◊ **Cholecystokinin (CCK).** A hormone that aids digestion and helps babies to relax and sleep.

◊ β-endorphins. Endorphins are natural painkillers. It's thought that beta-endorphins may help babies adjust to the stress of adapting to life outside the womb.

◊ **Parathyroid hormone (PTH), Parathyroid hormone-related peptide (PTHrP), and Calcitonin.** These help to regulate calcium levels.

◊ β-defensin-1. This is an antimicrobial peptide that helps prevent illness and infection.

◊ **Gastrin.** This aids digestion.

◊ **Motilin**

◊ **Bombesin (gastric releasing peptide, also known as neuromedin B).** Aids digestion.

◊ Neurotensin

◊ Somatostatin

Hormones. Hormones are chemical messengers that carry signals from one cell, or group of cells, to another via the blood. Studies on monkeys have found that hormone signalling through milk affects the feeding behaviour, temperament, and weight gain of infant monkeys. Hormones in breast milk include:

◊ **Leptin.** Leptin is a hormone that suppresses appetite. This may help prevent overeating in later life, which could reduce the risk of obesity.

◊ **Oxytocin.** This hormone induces feelings of relaxation and well-being in both the child and the mother.

◊ **Cortisol.** This can help control blood sugar levels and reduce inflammation.

◊ **Triiodothyronine (T3), Thyroxine (T4), Thyroid-stimulating hormone (TSH) (also known as thyrotropin), and Thyroid releasing hormone (TRH).** The most important role of these thyroid hormones is to control how the body metabolises food. However, they also have a key role in heart function, muscle control, brain development, and bone maintenance.

◊ **Prolactin.** This has more than 300 functions in the body, including acting on the reproductive system and regulating the immune system.

◊ **Insulin.** This regulates blood sugar levels.

◊ **Corticosterone**

◊ **Thrombopoietin.** This is important for the production of platelets.

◊ **Gonadotropin-releasing hormone (GnRH).** This regulates and maintains the reproductive system.

◊ **GRH**

◊ **Ghrelin.** This stimulates the appetite to increase food intake.

◊ **Adiponectin.** This regulates blood sugar levels and the breakdown of fatty acids.

◊ **Feedback Inhibitor of Lactation (FIL).** A whey protein that increases in amount as the breast fills up. It tells the body to slow down milk production when it is present in high amounts and allows faster milk production when it is present in lower amounts when the breast is less full.

◊ **Eicosanoids.** These influence the immune system by controlling inflammation to help fight infections, and they can help regulate blood pressure.

◊ **Prostaglandins (enzymatically derived from fatty acids), PG-E1, PG-E2, PG-F2, and Leukotrienes.** These hormones are usually made at the site of an illness or injury; they control inflammation, regulate blood flow, and blood clotting.

◊ **Thromboxanes.** This is a substance made by platelets that helps blood clotting.

◊ **Prostacyclins.** These can help blood flow by preventing blood clots.

Enzymes. These are special proteins that speed up certain chemical reactions throughout the body. Some of the enzymes in breast milk include:

◊ **Amylase.** This enables the digestion of starch

◊ **Histaminase.** This enzyme inactivates and breaks down histamine, a substance that the body releases during an allergic reaction or times of stress.

◊ **Lysozyme.** This enzyme is found in significant quantities in breast milk. It is anti-inflammatory and kills bacteria cells by breaking down their cell wall. It's thought to protect against diarrheal illnesses and is particularly effective against E. coli and salmonella. Its concentration in breast milk increases as babies get older and more mobile and increase further beyond the child's first birthday.

Other enzymes in breast milk include:

- ⬦ **Arysulfatase.** This helps process sulfatides, a substance important in cell membranes.

- ⬦ **Catalase.** This enzyme helps break water down into hydrogen and oxygen and helps protect the body from damage by peroxide, which is constantly produced by various chemical reactions in the body.

- ⬦ **Lipase.** This helps with the digestion of fats.

- ⬦ **PAF-acetylhydrolase.** This mediates inflammation and immune response.

- ⬦ **Phosphatase.** This helps break down phosphates, which are important for the development of bones and teeth.

- ⬦ **Xanthine oxidase**

- ⬦ **Antiproteases.** Thought to bind themselves to macromolecules such as enzymes and, as a result, prevent allergic and anaphylactic reactions).

- ⬦ **a-1-antitrypsin and a-1-antichymotrypsin.** These help to protect the lungs from inflammation.

Antimicrobial Factors. These are used by the immune system to identify and neutralize foreign objects, such as bacteria and viruses.

- ⬦ **Leukocytes.** White blood cells help fight illness and infection.

- ⬦ **Phagocytes.** These engulf bacteria and foreign objects and destroy them.

- ⬦ **Basophils.** These help fight parasitic infections, prevent blood clotting, and can help mediate allergic reactions.

- ⬦ **Neutrophils.** These destroy bacteria and foreign objects at the site of an injury or infection.

◊ **Eoisinophils.** These are a specialized immune cells that migrate to the site of an injury or infection and kill bacteria and parasites.

◊ **Macrophages.** These engulf and destroy bacteria and release signals that alert the immune system to the presence of an infection.

◊ **Lymphocytes, B lymphocytes (also known as B cells), and T lymphocytes (also known as T cells).** Lymphocytes are cells that recognise proteins on the surface of pathogens called antigens. B lymphocytes produce antibodies. Each B cell makes one specific type of antibody, and those antibodies each "match" with a specific antigen. The antibodies and the antigens fit together like a key and a lock. When the antibody locks onto an antigen, it marks it for destruction by the rest of the immune system. Memory B cells can stay in the body for decades, helping the immune system to "remember" certain pathogens, which means the immune system can respond faster next time it encounters the same type of infection. There are several different types of T-cells. Cytotoxic T cells help protect the body from illness and infection by killing infected cells or tumorous cells. Helper T cells can activate other immune cells and help B cells to produce antibodies. Memory T cells are like Memory B cells in that they help the immune system "remember" pathogens it's encountered previously.

◊ **sIgA (Secretory immunoglobulin A).** This is the most important anti-infective factor in breast milk. Babies are born with low levels of sIgA. It gradually increases as they grow, but through breastfeeding, babies can receive an abundance of sIgA. It helps to coat and seal the respiratory and intestinal tract, which protects babies from a wide range of infections. It is also highly specialized to the baby's environment. The baby's mother synthesizes antibodies whenever she comes into contact with a pathogen, and these specific antibodies are passed onto the baby.

- ◊ **IgA2** is an antibody which plays an important role in the immune function of mucus membranes.

- ◊ **IgG.** Similar to sIgA, this helps to protect the baby from pathogens. IgA antibodies help protect the baby from bacterial and viral infections of the respiratory and gastric tract.

- ◊ **IgD** tells B cells to be activated.

- ◊ **IgM** antibodies made in response to infection.

- ◊ **IgE** produces an immune response when an allergen is present.

- ◊ **Complement C1, Complement C2, Complement C3, Complement C4, Complement C5, Complement C6, Complement C7, Complement C8, and Complement C9.** These are proteins in the immune system, which work to enhance the ability of antibodies and other pathogen killing cells.

- ◊ **Glycoproteins.** These enable white blood cells to travel around the body. They also have a role in helping the digestive and reproductive systems.

- ◊ **Mucins.** Attaches to bacteria and viruses to prevent them from clinging to mucosal tissues.

- ◊ **Lactadherin.** This binds to certain pathogens and prevents them from reproducing.

- ◊ **Alpha-lactoglobulin.** This helps essential nutrients absorb.

- ◊ **Alpha-2 macroglobulin** acts as a defence barrier against pathogens in plasma.

- ◊ **Bifidus Factor.** Increases growth of Lactobacillus Bifidus, which is a good bacteria.

- ◊ **Lactoferrin.** Binds to iron, which prevents harmful bacteria from using the iron to grow.

- ◊ **Lactoperoxidase.** This is a natural antibacterial agent.

- ◊ **B12 binding protein.** This deprives microorganisms of vitamin B12.

- ◊ **Fibronectin.** This makes phagocytes more aggressive, minimizes inflammation, and repairs damage caused by inflammation.

◇ **Oligosaccharides (more than 200 different kinds).** These are complex carbohydrates that are found in breast milk but not in formula or bovine milk. They intercept antigens, especially *Pneumococcus*, and prevent them from sticking to the digestive tract.

Protein. Protein is essential for growth and repair. Dietary protein also provides essential amino acids.

Fat. Fat is really important for babies and makes up about 50% of their daily calorie intake. Fat helps the body to absorb vitamins A, D, E, and K, and it is essential for neurological development and brain function.

Vitamins

C: Vitamin C supports the immune system and helps the body to absorb Iron.

A: Vitamin A is important for supporting the immune system and for vision and healthy skin.

D: Vitamin D supports the growth of bones and muscles.

E: Vitamin E supports the immune system and protects the eyes and skin.

K: Vitamin K is needed for blood clotting.

B1: B1 is used for turning food into energy.

B2: B2 keeps the eyes and nervous system healthy.

B6 : Makes haemoglobin, the substance in red blood cells that carries oxygen through the body

B12: B12 makes red blood cells and helps the body absorb folic acid.

Niacin: A type of B vitamin – helps to metabolise fats and proteins and helps the nervous system to work properly.

Folic acid: A synthetic form of folate, helps to build DNA

Pantothenic acid: Also known as vitamin B5. It is necessary for converting food into energy.

Calcium: Aids with bone development

Phosphorous: This is a component of bones, teeth, DNA, and RNA. Also, a component of cell membrane structure and of the **body's** key energy source which is called ATP. Lots of proteins and sugars in the body are phosphorylated

Magnesium: Magnesium helps to convert food into energy and plays a role in bone health and repair

Iron: Iron is essential for the production of haemoglobin, the oxygen-carrying protein found in red blood cells.

Zinc: Zinc aids in the production of new cells and enzymes, wound healing, and helps the body process carbohydrates, fat, and protein.

Manganese: Manganese helps to produce and activate certain enzymes

Copper: Copper helps the production of red and white blood cells and triggers the release of iron to form haemoglobin- the protein that transports oxygen around the body.

Iodine: Iodine helps the production of thyroid hormones, which in turn keep the body's cells and metabolism healthy.

Sodium: Sodium helps to balance the amount of fluid in the body

Chloride: Alongside sodium, this helps to regulate the amount of fluid in the body, and aids digestion

Potassium: Potassium keeps the heart working properly and regulates the amount of fluid in the body.

I hope that this comprehensive list helps to demonstrate the huge number of unique and incredible ingredients in human milk. We can't eradicate these powerful ingredients by giving baby some formula. Breastmilk works in a dose responsive way, meaning the more you give, the bigger the effects – but ANY is wonderful for your baby.

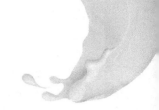

CHAPTER 5

The Benefits of Breastfeeding While Combination-Feeding

Studies that explicitly look at combination-feeding are hard to come by. However, there are a good number that look at formula-feeding and breastmilk feeding, and what happens if babies have more breastmilk vs less breastmilk. Below, I have added some summaries from a few of these studies that are interesting and, I think, reassuring.

Firstly, the study below found that ever giving a baby breastmilk helped to reduce the risk of Sudden Infant Death Syndrome.

> Results demonstrated that "ever" breastfeeding was associated with a reduction in the crude and adjusted risk of SIDS. The authors concluded that the risk of SIDS is 56% higher among infants who are never breastfed compared to "ever breastfed" infants. However, results for exclusive breastfeeding or specific durations were not reported (Ip et al., 2007).

A German study by Vennemann et al. (2009) found that while exclusive breastfeeding at one month of age halved the chances of SIDS. Even partial breastfeeding provided some protection. The authors concluded that exclusive breastfeeding reduces the risk of SIDS by 50% for all ages in infancy.

A 2015 study found that while exclusive breastfeeding reduced the risk of childhood obesity, receiving any breastmilk also provided some protection. They say in the study that combination-feeding is preferable to only formula-feeding in regard to obesity outcomes (Rossiter et al., n.d.).

A 2008 systematic review looked at 17 studies about high cholesterol in adulthood and how these adults were fed as babies. The outcomes suggest that babies receiving *any* breastmilk were less likely to have high cholesterol later in life. The greatest protection came from exclusive breastfeeding. (Owen, et al., 2008).

Antibodies

The breastfeeding website, Kellymom.com, notes the following.

> Research has shown that the benefits of breastfeeding are generally dose-related: **the more breastmilk, the greater the benefit**. But even 50 ml of breastmilk per day (or less – there is little research on this) may help to keep your baby healthier than if he received none at all. In fact, the immunities in mom's milk have been shown to increase in concentration as the quantity of milk decreases (https://kellymom.com/ages/weaning/wean-how/weaning-partial/).

Oral Development

Studies are a little unclear here, but one shows that while bottle-feeding did increase the likelihood of some dental challenges, this was nowhere near as important as what the researchers call "non-nutritive sucking." On a pacifier. They go so far as to say bottle-feeding didn't seem to lead to an open bite (Viggiano et al., 2004).

We know that when a baby breastfeeds, they are using the muscles in their mouth optimally so that those muscles can become stronger. Breastfeeding also helps to shape the palate and jaw, making dental problems less likely. However, it would be logical to guess that combination-feeding is still going to give the baby some help with their oral development. They will be using those muscles and having the breast fill and shape their mouth every time they breastfeed.

The other thing to consider here is whether alternative feeding methods, such as cup or finger feeding, might reduce the chances of oral development problems. A 1994 study discusses how cup feeding supports tongue movements closer to breastfeeding, lip tone, speech, and facial expressions more than bottle-feeding does. So, using a cup may support your baby's oral development better than using a bottle (Lang et al., n.d.).

Comfort

Affirmation

I am all my baby needs.

LUCY RUDDLE IBCLC

It can't be said too often that breastfeeding is only partly about the nutrition and hydration. The breast is a lovely place for a baby to be, regardless of how much milk they are receiving there. As long as your baby is able and happy to latch, then breast nurturing can be enjoyed by the parent and the little one for as long as it is desired.

What can a baby find at a breast?

- ○ The smell of the womb from the Montgomery's glands on Mum's areola.
- ○ The familiar sound of Mum's heartbeat.
- ○ The rise and fall of Mum's chest.

○ Warmth at just the right temperature. Breasts change temperature depending on whether the baby needs warming up or cooling down.

○ The relaxing act of suckling. Studies have shown that babies show less pain response when at the breast during vaccinations.

○ The sweet taste of breastmilk, which some people say tastes like vanilla ice cream.

○ Somewhere perfect for dozing off to sleep.

Please never underestimate the power of being at the breast for the mum or baby. It isn't only about the nutrition they are getting. It's about so many other incredible things.

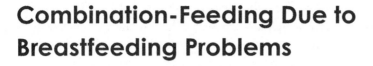

CHAPTER 6

Combination-Feeding Due to Breastfeeding Problems

Why Top-Ups Are Not the End of Breastfeeding

For many families, being asked to give their baby top-ups of formula feels like a huge failure. It's common for there to be feelings of grief or guilt around this, and that's hardly surprising given the underlying message feels like "you have failed to feed your baby adequately with your body." Add into this the way breastfeeding is encouraged—and even pushed all through pregnancy—it can be a huge shock to suddenly be told it isn't enough for your baby.

In the next section, we will spend some time looking at the reasons top-ups can be medically indicated because there are occasions where formula is absolutely needed. Goodness knows it has saved many lives *and* many breastfeeding relationships. It can't be denied, however, that quite often, formula is recommended when it doesn't need to be. That should be explored thoroughly to ensure that informed choice is truly happening.

The UK guidelines for supplementing with formula due to faltering growth state that top-ups should only be given while there is a clinical need. In short, you should be supported to reduce top-ups when the time is right, not left to continue indefinitely with no help to wean off of them (Health Development Agency, 2005).

You should also be encouraged to express your milk and feed anything you yield to the baby before giving them formula. (Obviously, this is where a return to breastfeeding is desired – if you want to carry on with topping-up, then you should also be supported to do that.)

For now, though, let's take a step back and a deep breath. We will take a look at exactly why you are not a failure if you have been told that your baby needs some extra nutrition in the form of formula.

Sometimes what we see is a baby struggling to breastfeed, leading to a reduction in milk supply and slow weight gain. This slow weight gain can then lead to the baby lacking energy, and the fatty buccal pads in their cheeks, which aid breastfeeding. The lack of energy and buccal fat pads can make breastfeeding more difficult for the baby. Then supply drops further. Before we know it, the whole day is one long, fussy breastfeed, and yet when presented with the weighing scales, the baby has only gained a few grams or has even lost weight.

Clearly, we need to help the baby to breastfeed more efficiently, and we need to help the milk supply to improve. Once the baby is well nourished, he will often have more energy and get better at breast-feeding again. Once Mum's supply increases, it's easier for the baby to feed again. So, we need to do two things: support the baby's nutritional needs and increase or protect milk supply.

If breastmilk from a milk bank or informal milk sharing isn't an option or something you want to do, then formula becomes the ideal way to support babies as everyone works towards breastfeeding more again. In most cases where formula is being given for slow weight gain, there is no reason why a return to exclusive breastfeeding is not possible with the correct help to get there.

Milk supply can go down, and it can go back up again. In fact, this is what it does during a growth spurt. Your body knows what it is doing. Formula does not often need to be a long-term part of your infant feeding experience if you don't want it to be.

Isn't that incredible?

Formula was initially designed to support babies who needed some extra help or where breastmilk wasn't available. It was designed for this very purpose. The commercialisation of it as a profitable product has meant that it's become controversial. When we see it as a medicine rather than a product, though, it does come into its own as a life-saving invention.

Common Breastfeeding Problems Leading to Top-Ups

This is important to cover because, based on the statistics, you may well be here after your preference to exclusively breastfeed was taken away from you. If this isn't relevant to your situation, please feel free to skip this chapter.

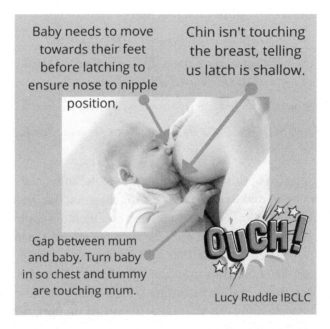

Baby needs to move towards their feet before latching to ensure nose to nipple position,

Chin isn't touching the breast, telling us latch is shallow.

Gap between mum and baby. Turn baby in so chest and tummy are touching mum.

Lucy Ruddle IBCLC

Positioning and Attachment, and Support

The reason people go on about positioning and attachment (P&A) is that it is the root cause of many breastfeeding problems. P&A that is just slightly off can lead to painful feeds, slow weight gain, low milk supply, mastitis, thrush, fussy feeding, frequent feeding, jaundice, dehydration, and rehospitalisation. So, if your baby isn't gaining weight well on breastfeeding alone, or your nipples are damaged, a breastfeeding supporter is going to want to watch your baby feed so they can see what the latch looks like, and what the feed looks like all the way through as well. We can tell a lot by watching a whole feed, such as:

◊ If the baby is held close enough to your body and in a position that makes latching easier for them.

◊ If the baby opened their mouth wide for a good latch.

◊ If the latch is shallow (we want a deep latch).

◊ If the baby is swallowing how we would expect.

◊ If the feed is painful for you.

◊ If any changes we suggest make that pain better.

◊ If the baby slips down the nipple or makes the latch shallower as the feed goes on.

◊ The possible cause of any fussiness during feeds.

◊ We want to see if Mum's nipple looks squashed or pinched after a feed.

Given this long list of things we can assess by watching a feed, and how tricky it can be to make sure you're getting it right alone, you can see why my first suggestion is to see someone qualified to support you. It is possible that you haven't yet seen the right person for the job. Often, people are surprised to learn that a breastfeeding counsellor, or an IBCLC, has a lot more training than the average midwife or health visitor in lactation support. Below are some rough guidelines for the training, scope, and experience that each type of supporter in the UK has regarding breastfeeding:

Peer Supporter

"More information about getting a good latch in the beginning would have been helpful, rather than relying on top-ups to ensure my babies were well fed."

~ Survey respondent

A breastfeeding peer supporter (PS) is someone who has breastfed, usually for at least six months. They are then trained to support mothers with common breastfeeding queries, basic positioning, and attachment, and to signpost parents to up-to-date and accurate information. Sometimes a PS is called "an informed friend." You typically find them in support groups, which they usually run themselves as volunteers. A peer supporter is so much more than someone with a little bit of training. These wonderful people are dedicated to helping those in their community meet their breastfeeding goals. They do so alongside providing a safe space, somewhere for babies and toddlers to play, and for parents to enjoy tea and cake or biscuits.

Peer Support Groups and Combination-Feeding

Many mums worry that they will not be welcome at a peer support group if they are using formula. The peer supporters should be well trained in understanding the nuances of infant feeding, and in giving the sort of parent-centred support, we sometimes call "unlimited positive regard." This means that you should feel welcome at any breastfeeding support group if you are mixed-feeding. If you are not made to feel welcome, then something has gone wrong, and it may be worth raising your experience with the group leader or the person who oversees the peer supporters. You are breastfeeding your baby. You are a breastfeeding parent.

If you feel anxious about going to your local group, it can be a good idea to call, email, or text the group leader, or one of the supporters, ahead of time so they can reassure you and know to look for you when you arrive.

Breastfeeding Counsellor (Inc BFN supporter and LLL Leader)

Like a PS, a Breastfeeding counsellor (BFC) has breastfed for at least six months, and in some cases, it may be required that she breastfed for longer–it depends on the charity or organisation the BFC will be training with. Typically, training takes between 18 months and two years, but again, this does depend on the training that the individual charity or organisation provides. You will also find a variety in the type of training from online with one-to-one practical work via the phone to classroom work and close supervision throughout training and beyond. A BFC can do everything a PS can: listening skills, positioning and attachment work, signposting, etc., and they can go into more depth for a lot of issues. They have a thorough grounding in breastfeeding education and are skilled at parent-centred support.

International Board-Certified Lactation Consultant (IBCLC)

An International Board-Certified Lactation Consultant is the highest level of training you can gain in breastfeeding support and is well-respected in infant feeding. The IBLCE (International Board of Lactation Consultant Examiners) exam is held twice a year all over the world. Once you have passed this, you need to recertify every five years through continuing education credits. Until recently, you were required to re-sit the exam every ten years. An IBCLC needs a minimum of 1,000 hours of supervised experience supporting breastfeeding families, 90 hours of lactation-specific education, and either a medical background or to have accrued 14 college-level health science courses to be able to qualify for the exam.

In the UK, many IBCLCs work independently, and this is referred to as Private Practice. This means they charge for their support. The reason so many are in private practice is because the NHS doesn't employ IBCLCs as standard in all their trusts. Compare this to much of the rest of the world where IBCLC support is common. You can see why independent work is often seen as the best option for those wanting to support breastfeeding at this level. However, you *can* find NHS based IBCLCs sometimes. They may be midwives, infant feeding co-ordinators, Health Visitors, or someone else who has put themselves through the training. Many IBCLCs, whether in Private Practice or working for the NHS, also provide free support services in the form of drop-in groups or by volunteering for helplines.

Finally, an IBCLC can help you with bottle-feeding as well as breastfeeding.

A Story from an IBCLC

A colleague of mine shared the following story with me recently and gave permission for me to share it. I have included their words here because they so perfectly demonstrate the sort of non-judgemental support you should receive when combination-feeding.

> I had an experience a few years into being an IBCLC that really helped me approach all families with an open mind to their individual situation. I was working with a postpartum family who had asked to see me at the hospital after their baby was born. They started off asking questions about mixing formula feeds with breastfeeding and how that might affect supply and latch, etc., but I could tell more was on their mind. I finally, gently, asked if they could tell me more about their individual concerns as that would help us create a feeding plan just right for their unique situation. Mom shared that she has a mental health illness and that she has learned to manage her condition extremely well with no medication as long as she gets 9 or 10 hours of sleep every night. She preferred to manage her condition this way and had worked hard to come off her mood stabilizers and antipsychotic medications safely while caring for her mental health. She knew she could go back on medications but preferred not to. Baby's dad was willing to do night feeds while she slept somewhere else in the home at night.
>
> We openly discussed their options such as pumping more in the day (which felt overwhelming to this family) and formula-feeding at night. This family, after a lot of questions and considering options, made the informed choice for dad to formula-feed at night and mom to breastfeed in the day. At the end of our consult the mom said she'd expected a lactation consultant would push "only breastmilk" to which I replied that I always strive to find the perfect individual feeding plan that feels right for this family in this moment. Breastmilk and formula are very different, but only the family can add the rest of the information on their unique situation that helps guide

us to what is best for them. We provide the information for informed choice. And then our job is to support that choice.

Some Positioning and Attachment Basics to Try

If you can't access support right away, these basic guidelines might be helpful. Please do also search YouTube for videos showing you how to get a deep latch.

1. **Make sure you are comfy.** This point is overlooked so often, but it is important. If you need to move around a lot once the baby is latched because your back hurts or your foot goes to sleep, then this can change the shape of the breast in the baby's mouth and/or cause them to slip or even pull away altogether.

2. **Lean back in your seat.** You may have been taught to feed with a straight back and a flat lap, but this puts a lot of pressure on you since you must take all of the baby's weight on your arms. If you lean back (pop a pillow behind your lower back if you need some lumbar support), then gravity will help to smoosh your baby onto you. Leaning back probably also ticks the comfort box as mentioned above.

3. **Once you are leaning back, turn the baby so all the front of their body is touching your body.** You particularly want the baby's chest and tummy touching you. If the baby is turned away, so there is a gap between both of you, they have to stretch further to latch, and this may lead to a shallow, painful feed.

4. **If possible, open the baby's arms so they are hugging your breast.** In a cradle/cross-cradle type hold, this will look like one arm on top of your breast and one arm tucked under your breast. Again, this helps your baby get in super close to you.

5. **Make sure the baby is lined up, so their nose is touching your nipple.** It might look like you've gone way too far, but

this position makes them tip their head back, so they get a deep latch.

6. **If it hurts, stop, and try again.**

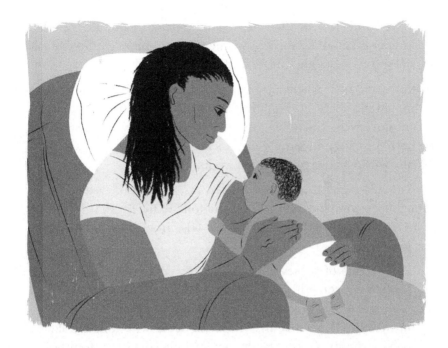

When having a look online for further information, try looking at examples of the koala hold and laid-back breastfeeding positions. Please get support as soon as you can if the basic information available here and online are not enough to make breastfeeding comfortable for you.

Tongue-tie

Tongue-tie is commonly talked about in breastfeeding circles. If you are having problems with breastfeeding, you've likely been asked more than once if your baby has been assessed for a tongue-tie. But what is it?

The lingual frenulum is a piece of skin under the tongue. It's considered a normal part of our anatomy, and the presence of this frenulum in and of itself is absolutely not a problem. What may be problematic, though, is if this frenulum is tight or short. A restricted frenulum can mean that the tongue can't move how it should move for effective breastfeeding. This might lead to painful breastfeeds for mum as the tongue won't cover the lower gum during feeds. The tongue is soft, and gums are hard. If the tongue can't extend out of the mouth, it can't massage the breast properly either. This leads to poor milk transfer and, over time, low supply. Other symptoms of tongue-tie include a clicking noise made by the baby while feeding, slipping off the breast, gassiness, fussiness, and messy feeding.

A frenotomy is where a trained practitioner uses a pair of scissors (or sometimes a laser) to snip the frenulum, freeing the tongue so that it can move well. This often, but not always, improves breastfeeding for both the baby and mum quite quickly – sometimes right away and usually within about two to three weeks.

I asked tongue-tie provider and IBCLC, Sarah Oakley, to share her thoughts on combination- feeding and tongue-tie. Sarah is incredibly experienced and well-respected in the UK, and I like the words she has for us here.

For parents of babies with tongue-tie, combination-feeding is often not something they planned or intended to do. Early excessive weight loss and/or the severe nipple pain and damage, or inability to latch at all, which can occur with tongue-tied babies, results in the introduction of supplements within the first week. Often before the tongue-tie has even been identified.

Whether a baby is given supplements to support weight gain, to allow the mother to rest and heal her nipples or to feed a baby who cannot take milk directly from the breast, expressing is key to protect and promote the milk supply. However, more often than not, mothers are not supported to express. Formula is suggested by health care professionals without any discussion about the long-term impact this will have on milk supply, and the mother's ability to breastfeed long-term or exclusively.

Prompt diagnosis and treatment of tongue-tie can mean that supplementation is avoided altogether or is only needed for a brief period of a few days. But if diagnosis and treatment is delayed, as is too often the case, combination-feeding often becomes a long term, rather than a short-term strategy. Mothers get stuck in a cycle of feeding at the breast, topping up with formula, and then trying to express to boost supply, leaving little time for anything else. The longer it takes for diagnosis and treatment the more likely it is that combination-feeding, or full formula-feeding, will become long term as this "3 stage" feeding cycle is not sustainable and parents understandably become exhausted and demoralised.

However, combination-feeding isn't always something that families fall into. It can be a conscious decision or choice for some. It may mean they can sustain some breastfeeding, which for many parents is important, not just in terms of health bene-fits, but also in terms of what it brings to their relationship with their baby and how they sees themselves as a mother/parent.

There will be situations where, even after tongue-tie division, there are persistent issues with efficiency at the breast and weight gain, or where supply continues to be sub-optimal. This may be due to early supplementation with formula or may be due to difficulties with expressing or physical reasons. In this situation a decision to combination-feed long-term may preserve the breastfeeding relationship longer term and so it is important that mothers are supported in finding ways to combination-feed that are sustainable and meet the physical and emotional/psychological needs of both mum and baby.

Feeding difficulties are emotionally and physically draining, and because of the difficulties parents commonly face with regards to diagnosis and treatment in babies with tongue-tie, the impact on mental health can be heightened. For some parents, combination-feeding will help to reduce stress and anxiety without the feelings of grief often associated with early cessation of breastfeeding.

Painful Breastfeeding

We talked about this under positioning and attachment. But sometimes pain is unrelated to the latch. For example, Raynaud's phenomenon or dermatitis of the breast can make feeding painful and may persist and, at times, be tricky to resolve. In some cases, it seems that despite excellent support, a few mothers continue to experience unexplained pain until the baby is older and bigger. If pain is an ongoing problem, it can be a good idea to seek someone like an IBCLC to work through what the cause might be and to see if it can be improved either with medical treatment or something more holistic, such as mindfulness, massage, or osteopathy work.

Dysphoric Milk Ejection Reflex (D-MER)

Dysphoric Milk-Ejection Reflex is something that still seems to be not spoken about much. It's a condition whereupon a let-down (or the milk-ejection reflex) the mum feels sadness – sometimes described as homesickness, irritability, or nausea. Mothers sometimes blame themselves for these feelings or think it's a form of postnatal depression. The cause of D-MER is not known. But given the timing of the symptoms, it is likely to do a malfunction of oxytocin, which is triggering a fight-or-flight response rather than more typical love-and- bonding feelings. The good thing about this is it tends to only last as the milk lets down. Once this stops, so do the feelings.

Some mothers find that D-MER is so unbearable that they want to mix feed in order to get some respite. There isn't a lot in the way of treatment for the condition, although we sometimes find that once Mum understands that it's transient, she might feel less bothered by the situation. Knowing that it passes as the feed progresses can mean that distraction techniques can help in the interim. It can also be helpful to note whether D-MER is made worse with stress, tiredness, or caffeine and for you to avoid any triggers where possible. Also, some mothers find that having protein at every meal can ease symptoms as lack of protein increases the insulin response, which could compound the feelings.

Sleep

So many families give a bottle at night because it seems to help the baby sleep longer. Babies want to feed often at night, and it can be exhausting to deal with this if you can't catch up on your sleep in the day. The Safe Sleep 7 is well worth looking at to see if bedsharing might be suitable for you and your family. Bedsharing was, for a long time, considered dangerous regardless of the situation, but more recently, we have begun to look at this more deeply. The Safe Sleep 7 sums up the requirements thought to make bedsharing a lot safer than accidentally falling asleep in the wrong place and at the wrong time with your baby. Many people write it off straight away, but I do recommend that you look at the information available first. In brief, the requirements for safer bedsharing are.

1. The baby was born at full-term and is healthy.

2. Mum is exclusively breastfeeding.

3. No one in the bed is a smoker, has had an alcoholic drink, or has taken drugs (legal or illegal), which could make them sleepy.

4. The baby sleeps on their back and is not swaddled.

5. The sleep surface is firm.

6. The room is an appropriate temperature.

7. Covers and pillows are out of the way.

Misunderstanding What's Normal

As a new parent, I thought my son feeding every 90 minutes was a problem. I thought that if he wouldn't sleep in his cot that I was doing something wrong and not teaching him independence. I wish someone could have sat me down and reminded me of all the reasons why a baby wants to breastfeed or be held, and that none of them are demanding, attention-seeking, habit-building, or anything else that could be described as negative.

Babies feed a lot. They do. And every 90 minutes isn't unusual. Tiny tummies fill and empty quickly. Mum's breast smells familiar, her heartbeat sounds familiar, it's warm, and it feels safe and snuggly. The act of suckling combined with the hormones in Mum's milk helps the baby to fall asleep. No wonder they want to be there so much!

Protecting Your Milk Supply If You Want to Exclusively Breastfeed

This is often an issue I come across. Parents being told to top-up but not being given clear, easy-to-follow instructions around how to protect milk supply. If we are replacing some breastfeeds with formula, supply will reduce. If the baby was feeding ineffectively and this led to top-ups, then supply is likely already reduced and will only reduce further if top-ups aren't managed carefully.

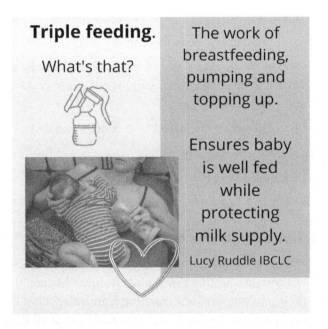

Triple feeding.

What's that?

The work of breastfeeding, pumping and topping up.

Ensures baby is well fed while protecting milk supply.

Lucy Ruddle IBCLC

Triple Feeding

Triple feeding is where you are simultaneously:

1. Breastfeeding.
2. Pumping or expressing your milk.
3. Giving the baby a supplement of breastmilk or formula, usually in a bottle.

It's called triple feeding because you are doing three different types of feeding. As you can imagine (or perhaps already know from experience), it's a time-consuming process and can, at times, feel utterly exhausting and endless. The road to reducing top-ups nearly always involves a period of triple feeding, in my experience. The key to making it work is often in finding little tips and tricks for making day-to-day life easier. These tips might include:

◊ Buying extra pump parts so you don't have to wash up so often.

◊ Hiring help in the form of a doula, nanny, cleaner, or a laundry or food-delivery service.

◊ Finding community help, such as a teenage neighbour, who might like to hold the baby for an hour, or play with older children in the home.

◊ Reducing expectations Mum might have on herself regarding housework, cooking, and socialising that she doesn't enjoy.

Expressing Your Milk to Protect or Build Supply

Expressing is often an effective way of protecting and rebuilding milk supply while top-ups are being given. Let's go over some top tips.

◊ Try to use an electric pump – double, if possible. Make sure that your pump is in good working order, preferably new.

◊ Pump after feeds for about 10 minutes.

◊ Don't focus too much on the quantity. Instead, notice if the baby is happier at the breast for longer after several days or if they are taking less top-up.

◊ Hands-on expressing. First spoken about by Jane Morton at Stanford University, this can increase the amount of milk you get at each pumping session.

◊ The more times you can express, the more milk your body will begin to produce.

Other Ways of Protecting or Improving Milk Supply

Switch Feeding

This is where you repeatedly swap breasts during feeds so that the baby may go to each side three or four times over the course of a feed. To switch nurse, you would allow baby to feed from one breast until they begin to fall asleep/appear fussy/pull off. Then you would offer the second breast, switching backward and forwards until the baby no longer stays on either breast.

Breast Compressions

This is where you apply pressure to the breast to help the baby take in more milk. Your hand is gently pushing milk out of the breast while the baby is pulling it out. To do this, you simply push into your breast tissue and hold. If it works, you will notice your baby begins to swallow again. Maintain the gentle pressure until the baby stops swallowing and then move your hand somewhere else on your breast. Make sure to only start compressions if your baby is not swallowing to start with, and don't compress too close to the areola as this may change the shape of your breast in the baby's mouth, causing the latch to shift and become shallow.

Other Suggestions

- ◊ Offer one extra feed a day.
- ◊ Keep your baby with you and offer the breast as often as you possibly can. (This may not be appropriate with slow weight gain.)

> Good breastfeeding support to ensure positioning and attachment are correct is essential for your long-term success.

Drugs and Herbs

In some cases, you might want to consider something called a galactogogue. This is an herb or medication that helps increase your milk supply. While some have anecdotal evidence, some are backed up with science. I will list a few below, but it is always essential that you do your own in-depth research. Just because an herb is natural, it does **not** mean it is safe for everyone, including your baby. Also, check for any contraindications regarding the medication you are taking. The info in this book is for information purposes only.

Fenugreek

Fenugreek is the go-to herb for many breastfeeding families, but it does have significant cautions to be aware of. Importantly, there are no formal studies regarding the effectiveness of fenugreek, according to the Drugs in Breastmilk Information Service.

Two to three capsules, three times a day, is the recommended dose according to most sources. It's worth noting that the amount of fenugreek present in teas is probably much, much lower than the amounts suggested. Kellymom.com discusses the effective dosage as being up to 2,400 mg a day (https://kellymom.com/bf/can-i-breastfeed/herbs/fenugreek/).

As already mentioned, there are some risks associated with fenugreek, including:

- ⬡ It's an anticoagulant effect, making it contraindicated if the mother is at risk of any bleeding disorders.
- ⬡ Contraindicated if Mum is using NSAIDs.
- ⬡ Increased risk of miscarriage.
- ⬡ Can cause nausea, vomiting, and diarrhoea.
- ⬡ May worsen asthma.
- ⬡ Can increase the risk of dehydration for Mum.
- ⬡ May cause hypotension or dizziness.
- ⬡ Increases the risk of hypoglycaemia, especially in diabetics.

Goat's Rue

According to Lactmed (Drugs and Lactation Database), goat's rue has been used all around the world to increase milk supply, but as is common with herbal galactagogues, valid studies to support its use are in short supply. There are a few old and poorly designed studies that suggest that goat's rue can be helpful for milk supply, but we just can't be sure how effective it is.

Dosage instructions are often vague and undisclosed in studies. Still, I did find one study citing 100 mg of goat's rue was given to mothers three times a day in a tea containing a mix of galactagogue herbs, and all of the mothers drinking this tea produced more milk with a pump compared to their peers who weren't drinking the tea. As this tea included many other galactagogues, including fenugreek, we can't be sure which ingredient helped. Still, for the purpose of dosage, this study may be helpful when considering goat's rue (Turkyilmaz et al., 2011).

Blessed Thistle

Again, according to Lactmed, while blessed thistle is widely used as a galactagogue, there are no scientifically valid studies to support its use for increasing milk supply. Risks include nausea and vomiting and potential allergy to the herb. I could not find official guidance or studies suggesting an appropriate dose.

Moringa

Moringa is a galactagogue well-known in the Philippines and is one of the few herbs where there is a degree of sensible data to support its use. A 2013 systematic review looked at five small randomised-controlled trials for moringa as a galactagogue. The outcome was that while the studies were small and some cases not of the best design, moringa use was consistently linked to a greater milk volume. In addition to this, no adverse effects were reported for either the mothers or the babies in any of the trials reviewed.

As with most of the herbs I discuss here, there doesn't seem to be a universally agreed dosage. The best source I could find was from drugs.com, which cited a study where pumping mothers were given 250 mg of moringa in a capsule while their peers were given a placebo. The mothers taking moringa had a 180% increase in milk yield on day 5, compared to the placebo group that had an increase of 38%.

Domperidone and Metoclopramide

These are the two most commonly prescribed drugs for increasing milk supply. They both come with risks and advantages. Of the two, domperidone is usually preferred as it may be more effective, and its side effects are less common.

Getting either domperidone or metoclopramide prescribed can be challenging. They are off-license drugs for lactation. Doctors in the UK were asked to avoid prescribing domperidone following a study demonstrating a link between extended use and heart problems. Unfortunately for our cause, this study was carried out on elderly men with underlying medical conditions – not young, fit, healthy mothers, and it was at a much higher dose than would be used to increase milk supply (Van Noord et al, 2010). Despite the calls for caution, some GPs will consider prescribing domperidone if you're struggling with your milk supply. So it is worth talking to them to see if this might be a suitable option for you.

Lactogenic Foods

Throughout history, certain foods have been used to support mothers with their milk supply. We have little evidence to back up their use, but as long as you enjoy them and are not allergic to them, then they won't usually cause harm and *may* be helpful. Lactogenic foods include:

◊ Spinach	◊ Dried apricots	◊ Garlic
◊ Sweet potato	◊ Oats	◊ Barley
◊ Coconut milk	◊ Almonds	◊ Spirulina

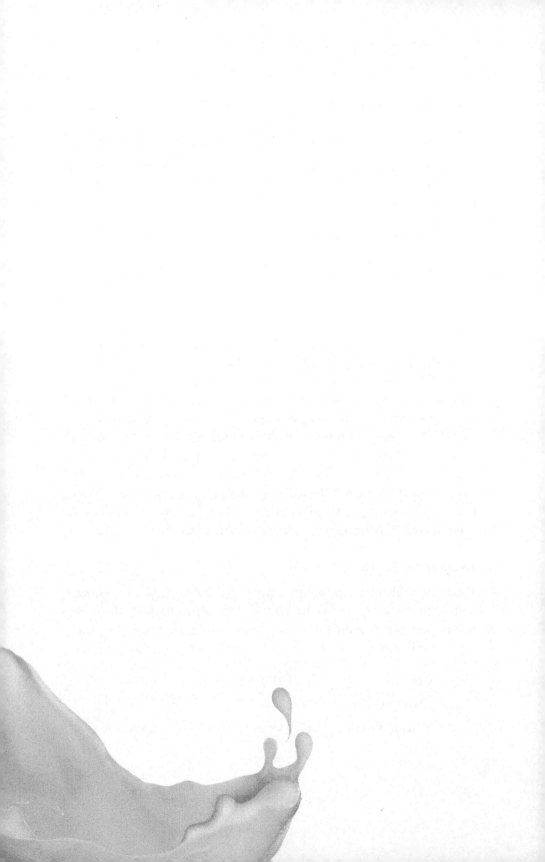

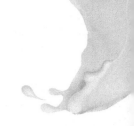

CHAPTER 7

All Things Top-Up

Reducing Top-Ups

We can often feel stuck once top-ups start. It can seem as though this is never going to get better, which can be a difficult place to be emotionally. However, reducing top-ups can be done, and I have supported plenty of parents to do so. The key is often to take things slowly, knowing that the process might take several weeks. This risk of reducing supplements too quickly is that babies might struggle to maintain weight, and Mum's supply could drop, landing the dyad right back where they started.

I discussed the following methods in my first book, *Relactation*, and I have added them here because they are so relevant. It seems a bit daft to rewrite something that already exists in my own words!

Bottle Sandwich

This is where we sandwich a bottle feed in between breastfeeds. You essentially offer the baby both breasts and then offer the bottle. (Paced feeding is *important* for this method. Otherwise, the baby will down the entire bottle regardless of hunger.) Once the baby has had the amount of milk in the bottle, you offer each breast again. As you go along, the goal is to reduce the amount of milk given in the bottle a little bit at a time – say 10 ml per feed every few days. If the baby is regularly leaving lots of milk, then reduce the amount offered by how much is being refused.

Finish at the Breast

Here, you reduce the amount of top-up by a small amount every few days – 10 ml is often suggested. You give your baby the bottle as normal but with 10 ml less milk in it than usual. Then you finish the feed at the breast.

If you have rebuilt a good milk supply, then this one is probably not right for you. But if you have a baby willing to latch while your supply is still low, then this is an excellent method to use. It will help to increase your supply further while helping the baby get used to at-breast feeds again.

Stretched Feeds

Assuming a good milk supply and baby latching well, you pick a bottle-feed to skip and try to only breastfeed until the next time the baby would usually have a bottle. While we don't rely on routines when talking about infant feeding behaviour, you have probably noticed that your baby wants a bottle somewhere around every 2 to 3 hours, or that they always ask for one at 6 am and 9 am.

Milk supply is often highest first thing in the morning, so you might prefer to start this method with the first feed of the day. The baby may well want to breastfeed often during your 2- or 3-hour window. This is okay, and you should follow his cues. Be prepared for cluster feeding (many feeds, spaced closely together).

Switch nursing can come in handy here. That's when you swap breasts every time the baby starts to pull away or fuss. You do it over and over again until the baby is satisfied. And it's a great way to increase milk supply.

If your baby becomes distressed and can't be settled with a breast-feed, then you should end the attempt and simply give the baby a top-up. If this happens, make a note of how long you managed to keep your baby happy with the breast and try to repeat that success the next day. Once stretching the first feed of the day is going well, you might then take the second feed and either try to skip that one or delay it by an hour or so. Simply repeat this until you are at a point everyone is happy with.

Using Bottles

Type

A quick internet search found me at least 18 different brands of baby bottles available in the UK, just on the first two search engine pages. These bottles mostly made one of three claims. Some made all three:

1. Designed like a breast.
2. Eases transition between breast and bottle.
3. Reduces colic.

As far as I could tell, none of these claims were backed up with scientific research, despite the great expense of a few of these bottles. Essentially, we can break baby bottles down into two categories:

1. Wide neck teat (shorter teat and a more breast-shaped neck)
2. Narrow neck teat (long, narrow teat, with the neck not much wider)

The advantages of each are debatable. We have little real evidence to support one type of bottle over another. It seems far more important that you feed the baby responsively (stopping when they are full, in particular). Some professionals suggest a breast-shaped teat is better because the baby has to gape wider to latch. Others feel that the narrow ones are preferred because it feels so different to a breast that the baby won't get confused. Whatever you choose, you don't need to spend a small fortune on a bottle that claims to help breastfeeding. None of them can prove this is the case.

Then the teats can be further broken down into flow rate.

- ⬧ Newborn flow (slow)
- ⬧ Mid-flow
- ⬧ Fast-flow
- ⬧ Vari-flow (The flow speeds up and slows down depending on the baby's suck.)

If you are combining breastfeeding and bottle-feeding, we usually suggest you use the slowest-flow teat available. This is because it might help avoid bottle preference, which we will talk about later.

If the teat collapses or gets squashed while the baby is sucking, however, it's a good idea to move up to the next flow rate or to try a different brand.

You may also see "orthodontic" teats – again, there is no evidence I could find to support their use over any other type. One comment I would make though, is, would you want your nipple to take on the flattened appearance of an orthodontic teat?

Paced-Feeding

You may well have heard of this. It's the method we try to use while bottle-feeding because it might help to avoid overfeeding. In addition, if you are switching between bottle and breast, there is a school of thought that pacing feeds makes the bottle-feeds more like breastfeeding, which means that the baby might be less likely to develop a bottle preference. It is also more respectful to your baby to feed this way.

How to Pace Bottle-Feed

◊ Instead of laying your baby back in the crook of your arm, sit him upright as much as you can.

◊ Offer the bottle by gently stroking the teat over the baby's lip and nose. When the baby opens, put the bottle in his mouth. Never force the baby to take the bottle before he is ready.

◊ Keep the flow slow initially by having the bottle angled so that only a small amount of milk can flow. You might be told this can cause your baby to become gassy or windy. There is more thought among infant-feeding workers that it's a fast flow and gulping, which causes more problems.

◊ After several seconds, tip the bottle a little, so the flow is faster. Your baby should have steady, unhurried swallows that don't look overwhelming. There shouldn't be gulping or spluttering.

⬦ If the baby is feeding a bit too fast, tip the bottle, so the flow slows a little.

⬦ Try to switch sides halfway through. This supports eye development.

⬦ The baby might take less milk than has been recommended per feed using this method. If weight gain is not an issue, then that's absolutely fine, and one of the reasons paced-feeding is helpful. The baby won't be overfull, so they should want to breastfeed again in a couple of hours or so.

⬦ If weight gain has been an issue for your baby, please talk to your health care provider about whether paced-feeding is helpful in your case.

Signs of Stress While Bottle-Feeding

It's harder for babies to simply stop a bottle-feed if the flow is too fast or if they are feeling uncomfortable. Pay close attention for the following stress cues that tell you it might be time to pause feeding, give the baby a cuddle, and try again in a few minutes if the baby does seem to still be hungry.

⬦ Gulping/spluttering/choking

⬦ Turning the head away or looking away from the person feeding them

⬦ Arching their back

⬦ Yawning

⬦ Hiccups

⬦ Fussiness

⬦ A high-pitched whine/whinge noise (Lauwers & Swisher, 2015, p. 521).

Hunger Cues

Regardless of feeding method, babies will show us hunger cues, and our job as parents is to respond to those cues as early as possible. When we respond to early feeding cues, we are doing our best to make sure the feed is relaxed for the baby and for the parents as well. Waiting until the baby is crying means we need to calm the baby down before they can feed, and this can take time. Babies struggling with breastfeeding may be unable to latch if they are hungry and might scream loudly or pull away from the breast when feeding is attempted.

Feeding cues:

◊ Waking up! If your baby is beginning to wake up, they are probably hungry

◊ Stirring/wriggling movements

◊ Hands to mouth

◊ Squeaks, whines, little noises

◊ Turning the head from side to side

◊ Trying to latch on to anything that is near their face!

◊ Fist or hand sucking

◊ Smacking their lips

◊ Fussing

◊ Crying

Try to catch your baby's cues near the top of this list. By the time we reach frantic latching, fist sucking, fussing, or crying, you will be more likely to find the feed is a hot, flustered mess ending up with a possibly unwanted top-up.

> **If you decide that a top-up is best because your baby is upset, you might be surprised at how little is needed. Just 5 or 10 ml of expressed milk or formula on a spoon or in a syringe will often take the edge off their hunger in my experience, meaning that they can focus more calmly on latching.**

Bottle Alternatives

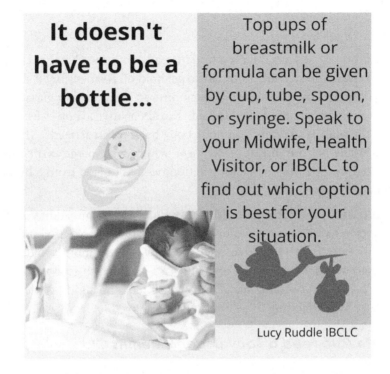

It doesn't have to be a bottle...

Top ups of breastmilk or formula can be given by cup, tube, spoon, or syringe. Speak to your Midwife, Health Visitor, or IBCLC to find out which option is best for your situation.

Lucy Ruddle IBCLC

Many families prefer to use bottles when combination-feeding or formula-feeding because they are familiar, easy to transport with milk already in them, readily available, and, well, culturally normal for us in the West. However, there are lots of ways to get milk into your baby without using a bottle if you prefer. There are some advantages to limiting bottles, including supporting oral development and tongue function, ease of cleaning, and in some cases, even affordability or availability.

You can, of course, mix feeding methods. Some people will use a cup or finger feeder while at home and a bottle while out, for example. If you're only giving a small amount of formula or expressed milk each day, you might find a teaspoon, or an egg cup, is fine. We can be more creative than many people realise. I will never forget one of my first ever home visits where I had the dad sterilising a teaspoon in a pan of boiling water so we could get some of Mum's milk into their sleepy 4-day-old baby. Where there is a will, there is usually a way.

Cup

Cup feeding is used around the world instead of bottles. Cups are cheap, easy to clean and sterilise, and easy to get hold of. As mentioned above, a "cup" can be any suitable vessel, including an egg cup, shot glass, or a spoon. They are sometimes suggested as an alternative to bottle-feeding when the plan is to transition your baby back to breastfeeds. This is because it avoids the "bottle preference," which can emerge as the baby gets used to the different sucking action needed to feed from a bottle compared to the breast.

There is a knack to cup feeding, though, and it's important you do it properly, as there is a risk of causing the baby to choke if you pour the milk into them. Of course, once the baby is 4 to 6 months old, you can use a standard open cup, and they can usually self-feed with just a little bit of support (and lots of encouragement and cuddles, because we always want feeding to be bonding and enjoyable) from you.

How to Cup Feed a Baby Under 6 Months Old

1. Get hold of a medicine cup (maternity units usually have them, and it's worth asking your health visitor too. Otherwise, the internet usually comes through. Alternatively, you could try a shot glass or an egg cup).

2. Sit your baby in an upright position on your lap. It's a good idea to wrap a muslin or a towel around their body to stop hands getting in the way and to soak up any spillage.

3. Gently tip the cup so the milk is at the edge of the cup and hold it to the baby's bottom lip.

4. The baby will lick or lap up the milk, like a kitten.

5. Do *not* pour the milk into the baby's mouth. This is potentially dangerous.

6. Watch your baby carefully for cues that she's had enough. Do not try to force her to take more than she wants.

SNS/At-Breast Supplementer (ABS)

Known as either a supplemental nursing system (SNS) or at-breast supplementer, this is essentially a feeding tube taped to your breast near your nipple, with a small bottle of milk at the other end. The milk flows through the tubing, and the baby gets milk while suckling at the breast. This can help to build your milk supply through the stimulation, helps the baby remember how to breastfeed, and can cut down on pumping time if you use it at most or all feeds.

The potential difficulties with an ABS are cleaning the tubing can be a nightmare as it's so thin. Furthermore, getting them set up and feeding the baby can often feel like it needs about six hands (when I used one, it took both my IBCLC and me to achieve a feed with it – in amongst a lot of giggling, because if you can't laugh when there's spilt milk and tubes and your baby's hands everywhere, then you would possibly cry).

When you come to buy one of these devices, there are two branded ones available: the Medela SNS and the Lact-Aid NursingTrainer™ System. You're looking at around £30 and shipment that can take a couple of weeks if you choose to buy one. You could, however, make your own in a way that is described below. A homemade ABS is a good way to establish whether it's a useful tool for you.

DIY At-Breast Supplementer

You will need:

- ◊ A feeding bottle with a teat (or without, if you prefer, since the only benefit of the teat is to stop the milk spilling if the bottle is knocked over and to protect the milk from anything falling into it).

- ◊ A 5 French feeding tube (NG tube) that is 50 cm long. These tubes have an open/close valve at one end.

- ◊ A syringe to clean the tubing with (5 ml medicine syringe is perfect)

Instructions

Make the hole in the bottle larger with a pair of scissors. Make sure they're clean – don't just grab some out of the drawer but give them a good wash first. The aim is to be able to push the tube up through the teat, with the tube's open valve at the very bottom of the bottle.

You may prefer to pop another small hole next to the larger one (with a clean and sterile needle, for example). This lets air into the bottle and means the baby doesn't have to suck harder as the bottle empties. This isn't essential, though, so feel free to experiment.

Put your milk carefully into the bottle and put the teat back on the bottle.

You can pop the bottle on a nearby firm surface or anywhere safe and close enough, even in between your breasts. A longer tube (for example, 90 cm) obviously gives you more wiggle room.

Place the end of the tube next to your nipple, so the baby takes it into his mouth as he latches. You could also try latching your baby first and then gently pushing the tube into the corner of his mouth.

You can alter the flow rate by moving the bottle higher and lower. The higher you hold the bottle, the faster the milk will flow. You might also want to try a 6 French tube instead as the wider hole will allow a faster flow of milk for a baby who isn't strong enough to suck through the smaller tube.

Instead of a bottle, you could use a 20 ml syringe. If you draw the milk up into it and then pop the plunger out altogether, the milk will flow freely into the tubing. You could even tuck this inside your bra strap, so you don't need to hold it.

It's important that the tubing is replaced often since they are tricky to clean properly and don't handle a lot of sterilizing well. You'll struggle to find a consensus on how often they need to be replaced. Different sources state anywhere from 24 hours to "a few days" if the tube is carefully washed after every use. As always, use your own best judgement.

Finger Feeding

Finger feeding is where you tape an NG tube filled with milk (like with the ABS) to the pad of your finger and use it to feed your baby. You offer the finger to the baby as you would offer a breast and wait for him to open wide before inserting it into his mouth. You then gently take your finger up to the start of the baby's soft palate and allow him to suckle. You can also apply gentle pressure to the baby's tongue using this method, which can help them relearn how to suck more effectively. It's a good idea to get your Health visitor, midwife, IBCLC, or similar helper to guide you the first time you do something like finger feeding.

When Your Baby Won't Take a Bottle

This is frustrating. You want or need to give your baby some milk in a bottle, but they won't take it. What do you do? Well, fortunately, there are some tricks that can help. Before we get into those, though, remember that you can try a cup or even a spoon to feed milk to the baby. Look at the previous section for more on these methods.

Top Tips for Getting Your Baby to Take a Bottle

- ◊ Practise! Try a little milk every day or two, in a relaxed, no-pressure way. If the baby won't take the bottle, no worries. Stay calm and "not bothered." Try again in a couple of days.

- ◊ Have someone else feed the bottle to the baby.

- ◊ Leave the house while another adult offers the bottle.

- ◊ Try having your baby facing away from the caregiver.

- ◊ Try having the milk cold or hotter than usual (but not too hot. We don't want any burns).

- ◊ Try a different-shaped teat. If you're using a wide-based one, try a narrow-based one and vice versa.

- ◊ Experiment with different flow-rate teats.

◊ If the baby is old enough (at least 6 months), see if they will hold the bottle or beaker and feed themselves. Ensure that they are sitting up and closely supervised.

◊ Try offering the bottle partway through a breastfeed or right after a breastfeed.

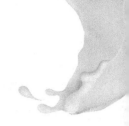

CHAPTER 8

Social, Cultural, and Identity Considerations

We live in a society that doesn't do a great job of showing useful and meaningful support for those who are breastfeeding. Many parents feel that breastfeeding in public is awkward or downright difficult. They may feel that they are being looked at and judged. They may fear negative comments or verbal abuse from strangers. For some, exposing their breasts or chest in public is simply not something they want to do.

We also have an expectation in society that babies feed every 3 or 4 hours. If you live with people who don't understand that breastfeeding is often an awful lot more than that, then combi-feeding may become a way to ease off some of the pressure from those around you.

Sometimes mums want to be able to go out once or twice a week and not worry about the baby while they are away. Mum may be returning to work, running her own business, or she may find that her mental health is better when she has some flexibility around feeding.

This book's remit isn't to discuss the rights and wrongs of our society and its view on breastfeeding. Rather, the goal inside these pages is to discuss the reasons why combi-feeding may occur and to support those who are using a mixture of formula or EBM and at-breast-feeding. If someone feels that combi-feeding is the right choice for them, then the reasons behind that decision, while relevant and perhaps helpful to understand, don't need a moral or ethical discussion here.

Younger Parents

According to the U.S. Centers for Disease Control (CDC), women who become mums in their teens are less likely to breastfeed than other women.

There are lots of reasons, but the most-cited ones are a need to return to education, nipple pain, and low milk supply (Tucker et al., 2011). Breastfeeding may make mothers feel lonely, trapped, or even more different than her peers. Combination-feeding may well be a compromise this mother is comfortable with. It's a conversation she might want to have with her care providers if breastfeeding challenges (physical and emotional) are proving difficult to overcome.

Single Parents

This category includes families where the partner is away for long periods of time, as such is for military duty. According to the CDC in America, around 40% of families in the States are single-parent families and have a much higher likelihood of being below the poverty line than their married counterparts.

If you are a single parent, you are more likely to return to work earlier, work longer hours, feel isolated, and receive criticism from others (especially well-meaning family members who may be providing you with support). All of this makes breastfeeding potentially more challenging, especially if it's already a struggle. It becomes harder to find the time to address pain or slow weight gain, both practically and emotionally. However, it may also be harder to combination-feed or formula-feed. Once we need to add in sourcing, paying for, preparing, and cleaning up after formula, it might be that you have even less time in your day.

It may, of course, be the case that you have someone around for much of the day or evening who can step in and help with the baby while Mum gets a break, or runs her business, deals with her other children. In these instances, where breastfeeding is stressful, the mum may find that introducing a bottle of expressed, donor, or formula milk does free up some time and headspace.

Partners

Partners often express a desire to help Mum by bottle-feeding. In general terms, if we're looking at switching an at-breast feed with a bottle of expressed milk, the mum may find that she isn't getting a break by the time she's pumped, and then pumped again after because her breasts are full.

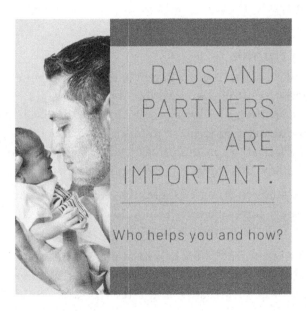

DADS AND
PARTNERS
ARE
IMPORTANT.

Who helps you and how?

For partners wanting to support, but where no one is sure that combi-feeding is desired or ideal, then there are other things that could be considered both to help Mum and to bond with the baby. Below is a list of ideas that partners and mums have found helpful.

- ◊ Wearing the baby in a sling and going for a walk.
- ◊ Cuddling the baby skin to skin so Mum can take a bath alone.
- ◊ Bringing the baby upstairs to Mum for a feed in bed when the baby wakes up.
- ◊ Reading to the baby.
- ◊ Tummy time.
- ◊ Baby massage.

However, if the parents have known from the beginning that they both want the non-lactating partner to be involved in feeding the baby, then combi-feeding may well prove helpful for both of them as they forward plan. Mum could express once a day, and over several days, her breasts will begin to settle for the missed feed. Of course, if formula is the preferred method of topping up, then breasts will also settle over several days.

Working Parents

In our modern times, many a parent will be running their own business or need to return to work while baby is still reliant on milk-only feeds. I discuss the options and practicalities of this in Chapter 2. This section though is a good space to talk a little about how maternity leave and/support to continue breastfeeding once returning to work differs, and how this impacts breastfeeding rates.

A 2016 study in America found that women who had at least 12 weeks of paid maternity leave were more likely to breastfeed. The figures were 87.3% and 66.7%, respectively (Mirkovic et al., 2016).

A 2018 literature review looked at 239 studies about maternity leave and breastfeeding. The authors concluded that longer maternity leave led to higher breastfeeding rates (Navarro-Rosenblatt et al., 2018).

In short, the more time you can have off work, the more likely you are to breastfeed. Again, I share this because knowledge is power. Combination-feeding, if exclusive breastfeeding upon your return to work isn't possible or wanted, may well be a fantastic compromise allowing you to provide breastmilk to your baby for longer.

You can help your body and your baby with the transition back to work by working hard and early on any issues you're having with latching or weight gain. Getting breastfeeding working well before bringing in a bottle or other feeding method is often incredibly helpful. Seek support as soon as you possibly can and set yourself up for success.

Pressure from Family and Friends

When our mothers and grandmothers were having babies, things were different. Breastfeeding rates in the 70s and 80s were much lower than they are today (28% in 1970 according to a rather sweet and interesting LLL blog *https://www.laleche.org.uk/rolling-back-years-seventies/*), and today's rates are far from good. Parents were living in a world where formula was normal, expected, and where breastfed babies were expected to behave like their bottle-fed counterparts. Routines and schedules were the way of the day, along with weaning at 4 months or often earlier. Parenting may have been more disciplinarian and also different from today in a huge number of ways.

All of these experiences mean that elder family members, in particular, are often baffled by "these modern mothers," as my Gran refers to us. Their comments about "Feeding again?" or about us "spoiling" our babies and children do come from a good place, even though evidence and parenting have moved on over the last 20 years. It can be easy to listen to your mum or your aunt, particularly if they're both sat across the table from you at Sunday dinner, declaring that your baby must be *starving* if they are feeding so often. It doesn't surprise me at all that mums decide to listen to their family matriarchs and give formula top-ups. The opinions of such relatives are strong and based in experience, even if that experience is often outdated now.

You might find that your family is open to learning about how things are done now, and there are ways they can access new, up-to-date information. For example, Wendy Jones has written a book called *The Importance of Dads and Grandmas to the Breastfeeding Mother*, which is a lovely, easy-to-read book full of good information.

The Association of Breastfeeding Mothers runs a course called Team Baby, which takes mums, partners, and relatives through normal breastfeeding behaviour. It's easy to follow and enjoyable as well as easy to access for most people who can use the internet.

Transgender Parents and Those Who Do Not Identify as Female

How amazing is it that we live in a more inclusive world these days? We are finally seeing open, public stories of the trans community starting families, and cases where non-binary people are overcoming physical and/or psychological barriers to providing their own milk to their babies. These barriers can be hard to overcome for a range of reasons. As an example, one person I spoke to (pronouns they/them) told me that having a baby at their chest and feeling their milk flow caused such conflicting feelings that it was too intense to exclusively feed from their own body. Combination-feeding formula and human milk provided a compromise that worked for both parents and the baby.

This is the ideal space to share Jacob's story. Jacob articulates the complexities of human-milk feeding as a transgender parent far better than I ever could.

> I'm a birthing parent to my now 2-year-old daughter. As a trans masc person (assigned female at birth) who has taken testosterone, my journey to parenthood was a little more complicated than most. I had to stop hormones to be able to conceive and stopping testosterone, which I'd been on for years, felt like stepping into a vast unknown. What would change about my body? Would I still feel like myself? Would my husband still love me?
>
> Despite my fears, I managed remarkably well and was relieved to find I kept my beard and chest hair even up to giving birth. The photos of me in the birthing pool show my still distinctly masculine body holding the baby I had just caught from my body and pulled out the water.
>
> Lots of things did change. My skin became softer and my muscle tone went down. My fat redistributed to my bum and my thighs, and I was suddenly able to cry again.
>
> What surprised me the most was that despite having chest surgery 6 years before giving birth, I lactated during pregnancy. Only a little but it gave me hope of being able to chestfeed using an SNS to supplement my milk.

When my little one arrived, I was met with a wave of dysphoria. I'd fortified during pregnancy but once my little one was born those after-birth hormones wiped me out and I suddenly felt surrounded by the word "mother" (which I don't identify as) whilst also being invisible as the birthing parent.

I withdrew from the idea of chestfeeding as I felt less and less able to even engage with the concept of my chest. I had the support of a specialist infant-feeding health visitor, and she was lovely and supportive. I actively wanted to feed from my body whilst also finding myself repelled from the idea. It was a shock to find myself reacting like that after I'd been so excited to produce milk, but I had to take a step back and focus on bottle-feeding my baby.

Regardless of how I fed my baby (SNS or bottle), we had always been hoping to use donated human milk. We used a well-established Facebook group to find people who had spare milk, and I drove all around to go and collect it in our trusty icebox. We even borrowed a spare freezer just to store human milk in!

We managed to use human milk for the majority of our baby's feeds for the first 3 months of her life. I found it fascinating how different milk from different people impacted her digestion and often wondered what different changes it made to her.

I mourned the loss when it came to feeding my little one with my own body but the one fear that I had, that we wouldn't bond as well, hasn't happened at all. We have an incredible bond, and I am still utterly amazed every day that I'm lucky enough to have her.

LGBT Parents

As the West begins to accept same-sex families more, we are also seeing an increase in the desire for co-breastfeeding to happen. I love this; there are certainly societies and historic references to communities sharing breastfeeding as their norm. I remember reading some years ago about a tribe where the children and babies would approach the nearest woman and just have a bot of milk before continuing with their activities. We're often quite removed from the idea of sharing breastfeeding in our 21st Century world.

Cofeeding aside, there are many issues relating to LGBT families and infant feeding, and combination-feeding may well be something that is needed or desired. I'm delighted to share the following from the wonderful B. J. Epstein, who has kindly written these words for us on the topic.

> There are many reasons why lesbian, gay, bisexual, transgender or otherwise queer (LGBTQ+) individuals/families may choose to combi-feed, and while some considerations are quite specific to the queer community, others are similar to why cisgender and/or heterosexual people might actively choose or be forced to choose to combi-feed.

> Many birth parents want their partner to be involved, and it is generally felt that feeding formula (or expressed or donated milk) through a bottle (or supplementer system) is one way of providing this involvement. What is different for the LGBTQ+ community is that for queer families with either two mothers or a mother and a transman dad or a poly group of parents, the non-birth parent may have strong emotions about their chest/breast not being the one to nourish the baby. Jealousy, guilt, sadness, or other painful feelings are all reasons for sharing the feeding.

> Some people have breast surgeries that influence the way they feed their baby and a queer-specific reason for combi-feeding related to this is the case of a trans dad who has had so-called top surgery. In this case, he may not have enough chest tissue left to exclusively feed the baby, because this surgery removes

tissue and can reposition the nipples and areolae, and may also affect the nerves.

Some LGBTQ+ people choose to create their families completely or in part through adoption, and although lactation can be induced in the same way it would for heterosexual or cisgender parents, combi-feeding may be an appropriate or necessary choice here too. In regard to family creation, generally, there is a huge range of ways that people build families, and coparenting is an increasing method; this may mean that a baby or child is breastfed/chestfed when with one parent (or one set of parents) and formula-fed when with another.

Although there have been huge developments in regard to LGBTQ+ rights in many countries and LGBTQ+ people often have access to better health care and more understanding treatment than in the past. Unfortunately, this isn't always the situation. It is not unusual for LGBTQ+ individuals to feel a lack of support from those around them, whether relatives, friends, healthcare professionals, lactation consultants, and so forth. In addition, some LGBTQ+ people are afraid of accessing support or feel ashamed or worried about doing so because they do not know what comments may be thrown their way. Lack of practical and emotional support and encouragement can also be reasons for turning to combi-feeding.

Also, in relation to support, some LGBTQ+ people do not feel welcome at traditional breastfeeding support groups or cafés or parent-baby activities, or they feel concerned about going because they think heterosexual, cisgender women will not welcome them there. Avoiding such groups or gatherings again means that they are not getting the support required.

Finally, mental health issues tend to impact the LGBTQ+ community at high rates, which means that the breast-feeding/chestfeeding parent may require antidepressants or other medication. While many medicines are safe while feeding the baby, some parents may feel more comfortable with decreasing the baby's potential intake of such drugs by combi-feeding.

Medication, support, partner involvement, complex families, strong feelings: for both LGBTQ+ and non-LGBTQ+ families, these are all important considerations when it comes to feeding babies.

> **B.J. Epstein** *is a senior lecturer in literature and translation at the University of East Anglia, a writer, a Swedish-to-English translator, a breastfeeding counsellor on the National Breastfeeding Helpline, and a trained doula. She lives with her wife and their two children and two cats in Norwich, England, and she can be reached at bjepstein@gmail.com.*

Race and Combination-Feeding

There is so much to say about why race is important when we are discussing infant feeding, and it is absolutely relevant to the topic of combi-feeding. This section was kindly written by Leah C. De Shay. BA: Psyc & SLP, CLEC, CMIc, IBCLC. I am delighted that someone so informed on this important issue has been able to contribute.

Here comes the part of breast, bottle, and alternative infant feeding that everyone wants to hear about, but no one wants to discuss: race. Along with culture and status, there is hardly a predictor more accurate (besides biological sex itself) that exists as a larger influence on pregnancy or postpartum experiences (as well as how their attempts at feeding their baby will go) than someone's racial and ethnic identity.

Now this topic of combination-feeding in the context of race deserves a few books of its own. However, for the sake of brevity, let's review how the intersections of race and ethnic identity directly impact and skew the likelihood and longevity of alternative breastfeeding and pumping experiences.

There are many admirable sources that cover the background of this issue (and we will refer to some them as sources and for future additional reading), but here we will be concentrate on something specific: the value and urgency of closing the gap between reported research and nuanced parental experiences with combination-feeding, specifically as it relates to race.

In the birthing field, doulas, midwives and other advocates who have stayed current on civil rights and reproductive research are aware that the difference in outcomes for birth and breast-feeding (and pregnancy and postpartum death) rates are due not to the racial identity of those who are of African descent, but the fact that they are treated differently because their race.

Likewise, the public health and medical community has since found out that no amount of socioeconomic nor educational increases improve the outcome for Black babies or birthing parents that are caused by racism (John, 2021; White, 2020). Unfortunately, the bias with which they are both unfairly perceived and treated by society and those who are supposed to serve them, remains so profound that no personal nor collective increase in social status or wealth has overcome it. Not that it should; being poor should never be a curse to eternal suffering, though it too often is. However, due to how much worse one is too often treated when poor and dark skinned, it is not only a curse but a death sentence, whether by prejudiced intention or biased neglect. Unfortunately, this speaks not of the power of race to affect one's birthing health and safety, but rather, the horrific threat of racism to overpower attempts to alter it.

This means the experience itself of being dark skinned in a world that doesn't value it, is the part of the risk factors for adverse outcomes with breast and bottle-feeding. It is this part of the struggle that research has yet failed to qualify: the lived experiences of Black women, parents, and families trying to recover from (what are often traumatic and medi-cally neglectful) pregnancy and birth, while dealing with a world that does not welcome them, and breast + birthing care less accessible than most. This obscure phenomenon is called weathering. The definition of weathering in this cultural and historic context is how one's "biological age" is accelerated by being the ongoing target of prejudice, microaggressions, and oppression; this context, social mistreatment directed at race and specifically proximity to Blackness. The darker and less ambiguously non-white someone is in feature and complexion, the more they are the target of biased and irrationally cruel or neglectful mistreatment by society as a whole, but especially those who have identities associated with the most power or highest caste as the case may be. This makes the likelihood of women of dark complexion and kinky hair texture more likely to show symptoms of long-term stress, including but not limited to physiological inflammation, chronic physical pain, insomnia or excess fatigue, indigestion, anxiety, obsessive compulsive disorders, depression, and the like. Despite this being a result of enduring racism all of their lives, they are also most likely to be blamed for the very conditions caused by their oppression; this is called gaslighting, and accumulated cortisol from stress literally takes years off of life expectancy in addition to everything else (Scott et al., 2019). In the most innocent corners of Western society (wherever those are), the drastic hormonal and physical changes alone can alter even the most privileged birthing parents mental and emotional state. Sadly, this experience and effect is extended to children—even babies—in utero of the birthing people trying to survive this social stress. It has even been found that the higher levels of premature birthdates and labor in both Black UK and U. S. populations is affected by this (Lane, 2020). How much more challenging does it make the transition for women who hold identities that society already overloads?

With that in mind, when it comes to combi-feeding, besides the basic statistics—which are now well advertised regarding the effects of racism on increased risk for Black and BIPOC infants and parents in gestation, birth, and postpartum—we must discuss the gap in care and support (both communally and medically) where ethnically respectful, and culturally fluent care should be present and readily accessible, but is not (Allers, 2017). This is not limited, for instance, to providers who find it appropriate to disparage Black mothers with stereotypical, false tropes about their identities or nurses who consistently offer formula while neglecting to offer any empathic education of any kind, but also extends to biased treatment by employers when they return to work, or having to return to school or work earlier in the first place because maternity leave is not economically stable enough or in places like the U. S., unavailable at all.

Twenty years ago, when research done by providers who looked and lived nothing like the communities they were researching, created (biased) results assuming lack of education would close the gap, providers ignorantly assumed that just because their present statistics showed associations between less breastfeeding and pumping or bottle-feeding, that the only answer to that was to eliminate both those options altogether. This was a false conclusion that has back-fired greatly. Interestingly enough, when "experts" wouldn't budge on the matter of "Breast being best" and "Boob or Bust," advocates among diverse doulas emerged to find ways to meet babies need for immunologic and bonding support of breast, while still supporting mothers need for sustainable options. We have since found out that not only can long-term primary or exclusive pumping be successful, but with the correct, empathic support, it can not only fully feed one baby successfully, but support entire communities needs for milk sharing as well. On top of that, long-term pumpers are the foundation and cornerstones of Milk Banks, whose survival NICU babies depend on (Meier, 2019). Exclusive and primary pumpers make lemon out of lemonade, many of whom are BIPOC women, trying to make the best of oppressed circumstances (lack of access to care, lack of support at work or school, neglectful providers who don't help with breastfeeding pain or tongue-ties, financial inability to pay) end up not only providing a wonderful alternative for their babies but also a life force for many others by becoming super donors who have yet to be thanked as such.

Those who have successfully combi-fed (breast and bottle (or any other technology, such as SNS or the like)) for extended periods of time, have proven to a stubborn, close minded community of breastfeeding professionals that with the correct oral exercises, habit, and developmental support, that babies can simultaneously support sucking skills at breast and with breast alternatives and go on to manage more than one method of feeding for as long as their parents desires. Contrary to popular belief, this should not be a point of conflict or controversy, but of liberation and relief. Nothing is more encouraging than finding out that when one's best attempts at breastfeeding go unexpectedly, that persistence will pay off more than perfection in the long run. This makes my favorite phrase, "Every drop counts" a reality that struggling, oppressed, and stressed mothers can realize for themselves.

There is no group of women and femme-identified parents who this level of understanding, diversity, and expertise is more valuable to in helping them realize and believe that every drop counts than BIPOC women. Statistically more likely to face anxiety, depression, insomnia, financial mistreatment, overwork, underpay, and lack of adequate access to support at home (not because their families do not love them but because they are all over worked and weathered in their community as well), they are the group for whom *any* intervention and creative care plans that are most sustainable are the most valuable. If after education and encouragement for exclusive breastfeeding is found to be inaccessible or undesirable, but sole access to breastfeeding is still desired, it is the infant feeding, maternal/child health professionals' responsibility to support BIPOC women completely. By showing humility, competence, and compassion, culturally and clinically, thus creating a consistent, flexible, reliable and sustainable care plan that makes maintaining whatever breast function they find reasonable, for as long as they desire to do so a reality. The barrier to normalizing and providing racially respectful, patient-centered care is not the birthing parents perceived complications or lifestyle imperfections, but the providers lack of expertise, compassion, cultural fluency and follow through, and it needs to be dealt with that way in order for things to change.

Patients can combi-feed for *years* with the right support. The problem is, because of stigmatization of working mothers, single parents, and really any family circumstances not popularized from lactation and breastfeeding organizations still stuck in the 1950s, too many experts either do not have adequate training or experience to provide the support, or when they do, it is so biased and judgmental, that the intended audience no longer wants it anymore. This is doing a great injustice to mothers who could maintain a less than "perfect" but perfectly sustainable amount of breastfeeding or pumping, and forcing them to move from exclusive breastfeeding to exclusive formula-feeding when that is not their desire. For this, an entire generation of parents and babies suffers: some breastfeeding or breastmilk is always better than none. As many a new parent will attest, however, most diehard breastfeeding advocates do not treat their birthing patients and clientele as if they believe that though; for the sake of not only infants but the mental health of their parents, that needs to change, both logistically and statistically (Da Silva Tanganhito et al., 2020).

Mathematically, if one parent breastfeeds exclusively for 6 weeks and has such a negative, exhausting, or traumatic experience that they quit, how much more milk would that baby have gotten if they had had compassionate intervention to combifeed, let's say 50/50, for 6 months? If we assume every feed is 2.5 oz at minimum, 35 min a feed, an average of 8 times a day, both breasts, 6 weeks of exclusive would yield approximately 840 oz and 196 hours of skin-to-skin, feeding time. For a baby fed 50/50 for 6 months, it is twice that: 1680 oz, and nearly 400 hours at breast. The difference is that this is spread out over more of the babies' developmental time. This means that it's seeding the microbiome of the gut for longer, and affecting the neurological development more profoundly over time than 6 weeks would. Is this "better" than exclusive breastfeeding? Not in the most trite sense of the word. Pragmatically, however, if it is a more pleasant experience for parent and baby, it is definitely an argument for a greater biological advantage and likelihood of sustainable success, than a parent who is trying to meet an ideal that stresses them out to begin with.

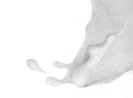

CHAPTER 9

Making Combi-Feeding Work

Consistency

If we think back to how breastfeeding works (demand and supply), then we know that the body can adjust well to a change in demand. It also makes sense that being consistent with when the baby has formula is a good idea, so the breasts get the message quickly about how much milk is needed when. This consistency could be that the baby gets a certain amount of top-up after six feeds a day. They might get one bottle at bedtime, or maybe three bottles a day evenly spread out every 8 hours. It might even be that the baby has one bottle a week or every few days. It doesn't need to be rigid, and giving an occasional bottle doesn't always need to be at the same time or on the same day of the week.

It can be helpful for daily bottles to be about the same time of day, though, as this will help your milk supply to work out what's going on and adjust accordingly.

Responsive Feeding

This means responding to hunger cues *and* satiety cues. When we're giving a bottle, it can be tempting for us to try and encourage the baby to finish the milk left at the bottom, but this can override the baby's full signals, leading to overfeeding and all of the tummy trouble that often comes alongside that. One reason why we think exclusively bottle-fed babies are more likely to be obese in later life is because they are more often overfed as a baby than their breastfed peers. The hormone Leptin, which controls satiety cues, can be switched off by overfeeding, leading to a lifetime of being more prone to overeating.

Trusting your baby over and above the volumes written on the formula tin is a good idea. Using paced feeding is an excellent way to help them feel when they are full before they are overfull. When we pace a feed, it's easier for the baby to turn their head away or pause if they've had enough milk.

Protecting Your Milk Supply

Perhaps one of the biggest concerns when combination-feeding is maintaining a milk supply. While many people have no problems here, it is a good idea to understand what low milk supply does and does not look like.

Low Supply Is Not

- ◊ Frequent feeding
- ◊ A baby who wakes when put down
- ◊ Being unable to express much milk
- ◊ A baby taking a bottle after a breastfeed
- ◊ Soft breasts
- ◊ Not leaking milk from your breasts

Low Supply Might Be

- ◊ A baby who cries after most feeds.
- ◊ A baby that is hard to wake up a lot of the time.
- ◊ Fussing/whining/back-arching shortly into a lot of feeds, particularly if the baby won't feed.
- ◊ Less than two dirty nappies a day in the first 6 weeks.
- ◊ Weight gain of less than about 30 g per day in the first 3 months.
- ◊ Less than six heavy wet nappies per 24 hours.

Tools and Troubleshooting

Dummies

Dummies, or pacifiers, are somewhat controversial, and if you are combination-feeding, you might be wondering about using one from time to time if the baby still wants to suck after a bottle-feed. The first thing I would like to say is that your breast is the original dummy. If you want to offer the breast, the baby may well enjoy that, even if they've just had a big bottle of formula or expressed milk. You won't cause harm by letting your baby have access to the breast for reasons other than nutrition, and you may also enjoy the oxytocin rush.

There are definitely sometimes that a dummy might be useful, though, and as with everything else in this book, my aim is to present you with all the information so you can weigh up your choices before deciding what to do. So, let's begin with why a dummy might be helpful for you or your baby.

- ○ They may reduce the risk of Sudden Infant Death Syndrome, although the views on this are mixed.

- ○ Some professionals recommend a dummy to help a baby with reflux.

- ○ They can help if the baby needs a painful procedure, such as a vaccination or heel prick test, but the baby won't (or can't) latch on to the breast.

- ○ A dummy can buy you a few minutes for a car journey, or to use the loo or take a shower.

- ○ A dummy can help premature babies learn how to feed orally faster (Barlow & Zimmerman, 2008).

Some of the things to be mindful of:

- ○ If the baby is sucking a dummy but not a breast, this may contribute to lower milk supply, particularly if the baby is combination-fed.

- ○ The baby may happily suck away on the dummy and forget to tell you they are hungry. This can, over time, lead to missed feeds, slower weight gain, and reduced milk supply.

- ○ One study found that dummy use in first-time mums led to a shorter time breastfeeding overall, with mums more likely to stop early (Mauch et al., 2012).

So, the key to successful dummy use may well be to only offer the dummy after feeding and for the shortest amount of time you can. It's also a good idea to allow your baby to have as much time as you feel able at the breast, even if they don't "need" to feed at that moment. Grab some snacks, put your feet up, and enjoy half an hour (or several hours) with your baby snoozing, feeding, snoozing, and feeding.

Choosing a Dummy

You might be surprised to learn that there is more than one type of dummy. You will typically find two types. One is traditional, with just a standard shaped teat you will be familiar with. These dummies are often considered safer. The other type of dummy has what is called an orthodontic teat, which sounds scientific and fancy, but there are some additional issues with these types of dummy. They seem to change the way a baby sucks more than a traditional dummy does, with shorter sucking bursts between pauses and a different sucking pattern (Nowak et al., 1994). This is important because babies suck in a certain way at the breast, with longer bursts of sucking in a particular pattern. A dummy that potentially alters that more than we would usually see with a regular dummy might make breastfeeding more challenging.

Safety precautions:

⬦ To avoid choking, always check the dummy isn't wearing away, degrading, or falling apart.

⬦ Try to choose a dummy with no parts that can come loose and end up in the baby's mouth. Any parts that may fall off should be too big to get lodged in the throat.

⬦ Never tie the dummy to a length of cord, string, or ribbon as the baby may become entangled.

Nipple Shields

Nipple shields are another potentially thorny issue. Some people hate them. Others love them. Most of us who work or volunteer in infant-feeding support take a more middle-line approach of "They can be helpful in the right situation." I've decided to include them in this book for two reasons.

1. If you are combi-feeding due to pain or a shallow latch, then you may be using them or wondering about using them, and it's important for you to know how this may impact on the breastfeeding part of your feeding journey.

2. If the baby has become breast adverse from taking bottles, a nipple shield can sometimes support them to return to the breast.

So, what is a nipple shield? It's a piece of silicone that looks a bit like a sombrero for your breast. It has a teat that goes over your nipple, and this teat has a few holes in it for the milk to flow through. Nipple shields are often used to mask painful breastfeeds, which isn't ideal, but they are also used to help preemies begin to breastfeed, for babies with a high palate or a tongue-tie, and for babies who have become breast adverse. In these cases, their use can be helpful.

If you started using a nipple shield due to pain or are considering one, for this reason, I would urge you to seek support from a qualified breastfeeding supporter who is skilled in assessing positioning and attachment. In most cases, pain can be greatly improved—or even eradicated entirely—with a little bit of time with someone who really, *really* knows their stuff. If you simply put a shield over the nipple damage, you won't be improving the root cause of the problem. Furthermore, as pain is usually associated with a shallow latch, and a shallow latch often means that there is a degree of poor milk removal, you could end up with low supply, more top-ups than you want to give, or exclusively formula-feeding against your preference.

Some other important things to consider when using a nipple shield:

◊   Is it the correct fit for you? It should be comfortable to wear, not pinching your nipple, but also not too big for babies to take into their mouths.

◊   Does it have a cut-out section for the baby's nose? These shields are a sort of half-moon shape, and this little cut-out helps the baby to smell the breast while feeding.

◊   It can be tricky to wean off using nipple shields. Some babies will totally refuse to breastfeed without the shield in place.

◊ They *may* reduce milk transfer. Because of this, it is a good idea to pump after a few feeds each day during the first week of use, and to have the baby weighed at the end of that week, to ensure they are removing milk from the shield as well as they need to.

◊ Occasionally I have seen mums allergic to shields. This presents as a red mark around the areola and breast where the shield was placed and, in both cases I supported, the skin was sore and itchy. This is rare, but if the pain gets worse, or seems to be linked to the shield, then you should, of course, stop using them immediately.

Looking After Your Breasts

When combination-feeding, one thing to pay close attention to is how your breasts are coping. Initially, you may find that they fill up and become swollen, engorged, hot, or lumpy. It's a good idea to be familiar with blocked ducts and mastitis, and also how to treat these issues. I'll give a brief idea below, but there are lots of other sources for more in-depth information.

Blocked Ducts

When one of your milk ducts becomes blocked with a clump of milk, or is just overfull, this can cause a lot of pain. It often feels like a bruised area on your breast and will be hard. Sometimes you can have several hard areas at once, and you may have a small blockage. Or you could have a much larger one, perhaps forming a wedge-like shape over a portion of your breast.

Mastitis

This is where the blockage has become inflamed or infected. It may also be that bacteria have entered your breast tissue, and that has caused an infection.

Symptoms include:

◊ A lump or hard area

◊ Bruise-like pain when you touch the blocked area

⬧ Redness on the breast if your skin tone is pale

⬧ A taut, shiny area on your breast

⬧ Fever

⬧ Feeling unwell

⬧ Symptoms that come on suddenly

For both mastitis and blocked ducts, the most important thing to consider is milk removal. If you ignore the blockage, or decide to stop breastfeeding at this point, you are at significant risk of developing a breast abscess, which is a nasty condition often requiring treatment at hospital. So, rule number one is to keep the milk flowing until the problem is resolved.

Tips for removing milk when dealing with blockages or mastitis.

⬧ Apply heat before feeds. A flannel, wheat bag, or hot compress – whatever you have to hand. Some mums even immerse their breasts in a sink of hot water.

⬧ While heat is being applied, and then also during your feeding or pumping session, gently massage your breast tissue from above the blockage or sore area, pushing right down to your nipple.

⬧ Consider dangle feeding. This is where you kneel on all fours, and the baby lies under your breasts on their back. You dangle your breast into the baby's mouth and make use of gravity, plus the baby's suck to pull the blockage out. If you have a shower, it can work wonders if you turn that on and dangle feed in the steamy bathroom.

⬧ If it is safe for you to do so, anti-inflammatory medication, such as ibuprofen can be helpful.

⬧ If you have mastitis symptoms or if your blocked duct isn't getting better in about 48 to 72 hours, then please talk to your primary healthcare provider as a priority.

Breast Refusal

Breast refusal may occur when babies are being mixed-fed. The sucking mechanism required to breastfeed is different to the one used to bottle-feed. With a bottle, the milk also just flows into the baby's mouth without a huge amount of effort on the baby's part. If lots of bottles are being given, then milk supply may reduce, or the flow rate may slow down. The baby may then prefer the bottle over breastfeeding, which can be upsetting for everyone. Below are some ways you may be able to help reduce the likelihood of breast refusal.

- ⬦ When using a bottle, try to pace-feeding.

- ⬦ Always respond to your baby's satiety cues, even if there is still milk left in the bottle.

- ⬦ Try to breastfeed before a using bottle.

- ⬦ Breast compressions can help to keep the baby happier at the breast for longer.

- ⬦ Switching sides frequently (switch nursing) can also help, as the baby will always be getting faster flowing milk if you do this.

- ⬦ Try to offer skin to skin while bottle-feeding.

- ⬦ Make breastfeeding relaxed, snuggly, and enjoyable for you and your baby.

- ⬦ Standing and swaying, or bouncing gently on a birthing ball can help a baby stay at the breast if they are beginning to fuss. This can also help to latch them on.

- ⬦ Bottle-feed with the bottle as close to the breast as you can get it, so your baby still associates the breast with milk, regardless of where it's coming from.

If breast refusal does become a problem for your baby, you can often overcome it. You might need some good support from someone qualified in breastfeeding support, and it will take time. But many a baby has returned to the breast after aversion, including my own.

Changing Your Mind

The wonderful thing about maintaining some sort of a milk supply is that it is often a lot easier to increase the number of breastfeeds given per day if you feel that you want to do so, or if you see that the number of top-ups is increasing where you don't want them to. Your breasts will respond to increased stimulation, and many mothers have even returned to full breastfeeding over time. The more breastfeeding you are doing when you decide to shift away from top-ups, the quicker and easier increasing milk production will be. But that isn't to say that you can't shift the balance where more top-ups are being given.

In my first book, *Relactation – A Guide to Rebuilding Your Milk Supply*, I explored in-depth how it's even possible to return to breastfeeding after stopping altogether. So you, as a combination-feeding parent, have a good chance of getting things where you want them to be.

How you go about this depends on how many breastfeeds are happening currently. If you are only giving one bottle a day, you will probably find that by reducing the volume in that bottle by 10 ml every 3 to 5 days, you will be able to easily drop it and breastfeed exclusively with no problems.

If you are giving more formula or donor milk, then you will likely need express to help your milk supply increase. Ten minutes after feeds, as discussed in the section on reducing top-ups will be an excellent way to help your milk supply. Look at that chapter as the information in there applies to you perfectly.

If you are nearly exclusively formula-feeding, and you want to breastfeed more, then you still have a good chance of doing this. Lots of pumping and lots of support will give you an excellent chance of meeting your goals. You might want to go to one of your local breastfeeding-support services, call a helpline, or hire an IBCLC.

If You Decide to Stop Breastfeeding Altogether

Of course, for some reading this book, there may come a point in time where you decide that you want to stop breastfeeding and only formula-feed. Making this process as slow as is realistically possible means that you are at less risk of mastitis and the low mood caused by a hormone crash many women describe when they cease breastfeeding suddenly. Slowly reducing breastfeeding also gives you wiggle room if you find yourself in a situation where you want to pause the stopping process. For example, if your baby is poorly or going through a period of waking more at night. (Because lots of mums tell me that being able to offer a breast is a great "quick fix" for nights like this.)

Essentially though, the work of stopping breastfeeding is straight-forward – particularly where you have been combination-feeding, so your baby is used to formula and bottles. The simplest way is to choose a particular breastfeed (say late afternoon) and replace it with a bottle. Breastfeed your baby next time they ask for a feed to avoid your breast getting too full. After a few days of this, if your breasts are comfortable and the baby is settled with the change, simply choose another feed at a different time of day and repeat until either all breastfeeds are eliminated, or you find the "sweet point" of breast/formula that works for you and your little one.

Normal Infant Behaviour

One common reason that mums say they stop breastfeeding, or intro-duce a top-up, is because they worry that the baby's normal behaviour is a sign that they need more milk. This misunderstanding of infant behaviour might also lead to extra top-ups being given where you don't want to. So, let's go over some of these concerns below.

◊ **Baby wakes as soon as they are put down**

This can indeed be frustrating because the baby is deeply asleep on your chest or at your breast. You need a wee or just to stretch your legs, so you carefully place your baby down and walk away, only to hear the tell-tale grunts and protests of a baby asking to feed. How can he be hungry? You *just* fed him! You pick him up, he latches onto your breast, falls asleep happily, and you repeat the whole process for infinity.

What's going on? Well, put simply, your baby is hardwired to feel safe when in physical contact with a human body. Bonus points if that human body has a breast producing milk to settle into! A baby's brain is primal. The only parts working at first are the bits essential for survival. And your baby does not understand that his safety-assured brand- new crib, in his double glazed 21ˢᵗ-century house, is safe. His brain alerts him to possible danger when he is somewhere cold and open (which a cot or a bassinet is when you weigh only 8 lbs). The baby will wake and call out for help, and an adult's arms to keep him safe from danger. Your baby is very, very smart.

◊ Baby wants to feed frequently

Somewhere along the line, the message that babies need to breastfeed around 10 to 12 times a day, *or more,* has become "Babies feed every three hours." This is an entirely unhelpful way to look at things. Partly because a baby can't tell the time but also because breastfeeding is never just about how full a stomach is; remember other reasons a baby or child may want to breastfeed include comfort, pain relief, reconnection, and to sleep.

All the extra stuff aside, what *is* normal for feed frequency? Well, if your baby is feeding less than 8 times a day, they might not be feeding enough. If they are either on the breast, deeply asleep, or crying, and you are counting multiple feeds an hour for most hours, day in, day out, then that might also suggest the baby is struggling to get enough milk.

"Normal" could be that your baby feeds hourly for 4 hours. Then sleeps for 3 hours, wakes up, has a big feed, looks around for a bit, then feeds twice more before having another snooze. They might then want to be on and off the breast many times over a few hours before settling into another sleep, waking up alert, gazing at you (at 3 am, you lucky thing), and then feeding a couple more times before dawn.

Normal might also be that the baby looks for the breast every 2 hours. Or every 90 minutes. Or maybe they wake 5 times at night, and then sleep on and off all day, feeding another 4 or 5 times in between sleep and play.

As your baby gets older, feed frequency doesn't reduce, but the baby might feed for less time when they go to the breast. They are also likely to actively seek the breast if they are tired, scared, hurting, bored, or just feeling cuddly. All of this is okay. It really is. You cannot overfeed them, even if you are combination-feeding.

◊ **Baby isn't sleeping through the night.**

Ah, the myth of the "good baby"! You know, the ones who sleep 12 hours straight every night? I've never met one.

Think about it. You might be used to sleeping 8 or 9 hours a night (pre-baby), but it's likely that you recall waking up at least once most nights. Maybe to use the bathroom, have a sip of water, or to add an extra blanket if you are cold. We move between sleep cycles all night long, and we momentarily wake up and stir as we transition between these cycles.

Babies are the same. Except their sleep cycles are a lot shorter than ours, lasting about 40 minutes. Plus, your baby can't grab a sip of water, pull on an extra blanket, or pop to the bathroom. They may also feel unsafe if they can't smell, hear, or see you. In addition to this, tiny stomachs need filling often throughout at least the first year of life.

> Put simply, babies wake at night for many reasons and they need an adult to help them with all of these.

Growth Spurts

Growth spurts can be confusing or even worrying for new parents. Often categorised by frequent feeding over a few days, it's not surprising that these feeding frenzies lead to anxiety in Mum and Dad. The first thing to note is if your baby *always* feeds most of the day and is unsettled after a lot of feeds much of the time, then you might need more support. Growth spurts last a few days, and during these days, weight and nappies continue to trend as usual.

The best way to cope with a growth spurt is to stock up on snacks and water, get a good box set lined up, and settle into your sofa or bed.

Red Flags That It's Not a Growth Spurt

The following signs might suggest that milk intake is challenging. Please speak to your health care provider if you see these symptoms in your baby.

◊ Growth-spurt behaviour is happening from day to day for your baby. It's your baby's "normal" behaviour.

◊ You see a reduction in wet nappies.

◊ You see a reduction in dirty nappies if your baby is under about 6 weeks of age.

◊ Breastfeeding is painful for you.

◊ The baby seems distressed a lot of the time.

◊ The baby seems unwell.

◊ Parental instinct is telling you that something is wrong.

Introducing Solids When Combination-Feeding

In breastfeeding support, we often remind mums who are forced to mix-feed that once solids are introduced to her baby at around 6 months, she will be able to slowly stop the top-ups and maintain the breastfeeding, often going on to breastfeed for as long as she wants to. This is another wonderful thing about breastmilk – you don't need to stop giving it at 6 or 12 months. The World Health Organisation recommends breastfeeding for 2 years and beyond, for as long as the mum and baby both wish to carry on. This is because there is absolutely no known harm associated with continued breastfeeding, and there are advantages for both the mother and little one.

As solids increase, you reduce the formula being given but continue the breastfeeding. By about 12 months, most babies have stopped taking formula, switching to cow's milk or a non-dairy alternative, and in the case of combi-feeding, that non-dairy alternative might include breastmilk.

Reasons to continue breastfeeding into the second year and beyond include:

◊   Immune benefits. Perrin (2016) found that milk produced in the second year of the baby's life was higher in lactoferrin, lysozyme, and Immunoglobulin A. These ingredients all help to support the immune system, which is still developing in toddlers.

◊ A study in Kenya noted that breastmilk in mums breastfeeding their 1-year-olds provided up to 32% of their baby's energy needs (Onyango 2002).

◊ Persson (1998) states that breastfeeding in the third year of life continues to provide an important source of vitamin A.

◊ Babies breastfed for up to 3 years have been shown to have fewer illnesses, and when they do get sick, the illness tends to be shorter in duration (Mølbak, 1994; van den Bogaard, 1991; Gulick, 1986).

◊ Mums who breastfeed are less likely to develop breast cancer, and the risks decrease further for each year of breastfeeding (Wise et al., 2009).

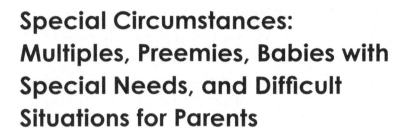

CHAPTER 10

Special Circumstances: Multiples, Preemies, Babies with Special Needs, and Difficult Situations for Parents

While much of the information in this book applies to special circumstances, you may not want to trawl through it to find what you need. This section will give a quick guide to combination-feeding your poorly or premature baby. This is not an area I deal with often in my own practice, so I am delighted that Kathryn Stagg, IBCLC, and Tessa Clark, RN, IBCLC, have added their valuable and wise contributions for you to read. This chapter will also discuss trauma regarding the breasts, particularly relating to a history of sexual abuse or body dysmorphia.

Becky's Story

Becky's story opens this chapter as it shows us that sometimes a special formula can make all the difference.

> I had a straightforward pregnancy and birth at 38 weeks and 1 day. My son latched on straight away, and we got off to a brilliant start with breastfeeding and went home the same day.
>
> On day 3 at home, our Health Visitor took a heel prick blood sample as my son was looking a little jaundiced. Later that day, we were called into our local hospital after the blood test showed unusual bilirubin results and needed to be rechecked. Unfortunately, the second test was no better, and we were told there was a problem with our baby's liver. Our local hospital contacted the nearest specialist liver unit, and we were told

that we must stop breastfeeding in case there was a metabolic problem. I continued to pump as I was desperate that this wouldn't be the end of breastfeeding for us.

We were transferred to the specialist liver unit on day 5, and I was continuing to pump throughout the day and night.

Our son became very poorly. His liver was failing badly. He was hooked up to all sorts of tubes and wires and was taking nothing orally. His nutrition was administered intravenously. On day 8, he was listed on the super urgent list for a liver transplant. Eight days later, a donor was found, and my baby underwent a liver transplant at 16 days old.

I continued to pump throughout this time, and for the next few weeks while my son was in PICU. He was still not able to take anything by mouth for the time being. As he recovered, the doctors were keen to introduce some EBM via NG. Finally! All the pumping was worth it. There were a few complications once the EBM got into his system, and he had to be put on a special MCT diet for a while until he was a bit further down the road to recovery. Another 5 weeks of pumping ensued. During this time, we were transferred from PICU to the ward. I had built up such a huge stash of milk in hospital freezers, and knowing we wouldn't use most of it, I donated most of it to the local milk bank.

With things improving well, the doctors were keen to try letting my son have some breast milk again, which thankfully this time didn't cause any issues. This was in measured amounts at first, so fed via NG or bottle. He would also have to have a prescribed amount of high-calorie formula to help him gain weight.

With things continuing to improve, we were encouraged to try direct breastfeeding. To my absolute delight, my baby remembered what to do! He latched on and fed like he'd been doing it since the day he was born. The doctors were all very impressed. They had encouraged me to continue pumping the entire time and were very active in facilitating us being able to return to breastfeeding.

We continued to combi-feed with the high-calorie formula, gradually reducing the top-ups until returning to exclusive breastfeeding two weeks before my son was 6 months old.

We went through something unimaginable, and I have no uncertainty that pumping and breastfeeding kept me going. I also have no doubt that it has helped in my son's recovery. Since his transplant, he had daily anti-rejection medication that suppresses his immune system, so the extra protection he's had from breastfeeding gives him a little extra protection. He's now 2 1/2, and we are continuing breastfeeding, and we both love it.

Premature Babies (written by Tessa Clark, RN, IBCLC)

For most babies, they grow quickest inside of your womb. When they arrive earthside earlier than planned, the increased energy demands of life outside your womb means extra calories, time to grow, and rest are needed to catch up. This often means a stay in the Neonatal Intensive Care Unit (NICU) or Special Care Baby Unit (SCBU). As a result, parents will have a different experience to that of those who get to take their babies home soon after birth. This adds an extra layer of complexity to feeding.

When your baby(s) arrives earlier than 37 weeks, they are classed as premature. This can be a worrying time for you and is filled with much confusion around feeding. I hope that the following information can give you confidence in the weeks ahead and empower you to advocate for your family and your personal feeding goals.

A stay in a Neonatal Unit (NICU/SCBU) usually means you and your little one are going to be getting used to lots of faces, information, and a new obsession with the life-giving fluid that is coming from your mammary glands. There will be lots of feelings, many negative, but none unique to just you. You are not alone.

Babies born before 32 weeks, or who are under 2 kg at birth, tend to be cared for in a NICU and sometimes might not be able to have only your milk right away. These babies are usually offered donor human milk alongside yours, as this is shown to be the optimal food for their developing gut. The risks associated with early formula use will be explained best by your healthcare team.

Availability of donor human milk for other babies in the NICU environment will vary from unit to unit. Please talk to your health care team for more info on your baby's situation and local policy.

The first drops of your milk, no matter how small, will be the perfect food for your early or sick baby. Even if you are unable to touch your baby, or are separated by different hospital environments, you can still care for your baby by expressing your milk early and often. This sets you up in good stead for a robust milk supply. You can store these precious drops in syringes, and they can be given to your baby soon after expressing or be frozen for later.

A rocky start to parenthood can mean struggling for a bit with hand expressing. If this was you, do not worry. Your breasts know to make more milk as you ask them to.

Once your milk "comes in," the hospital will usually have a pumping room where you can sit alone, or with other parents, to express your milk with powerful and effective breast pumps, which you may hear referred to as "Hospital Grade." There are things you can do to maximise your milk output, such as breast compressions and finishing your session with 5 minutes of hand expression.

As always in infant feeding, please remember that every drop helps. You *are* making a difference to your baby, even if you can't meet their full needs with your own milk at this time.

Emotions

Having a baby is emotional enough without adding illness or separation to the mix. Your emotions will likely be high, and you may worry you are not going to reach your personal feeding goals. The feeling of failure is common among NICU parents. While I cannot change these feelings for you, I can offer you some tools to keep moving forward alongside them.

Many of you may also have tools from antenatal education that can cross over into postpartum and breastfeeding. These are relaxation, hypnobirthing, and affirmations, which are increasingly popular. I shall lump these together into the term Mindfulness, which has been shown to increase milk supply and reduce stress. Lowering stress will enable you to be more present for your baby, whatever your feeding goals. The information throughout this book can help you with maximising your own milk-supply capacity. In particular, the sections on expressing, latching (when the time is right for your baby), and seeking further support.

For many babies cared for in NICU and SCBU, it is common for them to require additional milk supplements of Mum's own breastmilk, donor milk if they were premature, or a special high-calorie formula milk.

You may have been instructed to produce a certain amount of milk per day, and being unable to keep up with this requirement can undermine your confidence as a parent. Often, parents find themselves so worried about milk intake, even when things are going well, that they prefer to keep offering some bottles of formula or expressed milk for reassurance. This is not surprising given the pressure and fear that can be placed on parents during their NICU stay.

Many parents whose babies have graduated the NICU/SCBU will talk of the daily obsession with milk volumes, both consumed by your little one or produced by the lactating parent. This is likely to continue for some time after you bring your babies home from the hospital as you are used to it. Please know it is possible to transition into a rhythm free from numbers and clock watching with the right support and information, even with combination-feeding.

Very early and very sick babies are often too poorly to have milk at first, and sometimes you may experience a delay in your milk coming in too.

The sooner you can do this after birth, the more signals to your brain are sent for a full milk supply.

Your body will make milk that is higher in fat and immune factors for your baby, so even if your baby qualifies for donor human milk, yours is the freshest and most tailor-made that is available. Your milk could be viewed as an excellent medicine for your baby, so getting as much to them as possible will likely be encouraged by the NICU staff. Every drop is magical, no matter how much you make. Staff within the unit will help you with first feeds and work out volumes of milk needed in the early days and weeks.

First Feeds at the Breast

Premature babies tend to be able to breastfeed around 34 weeks as the brain develops. There are many babies who will show signs readiness earlier and later. Poorly babies and those with issues like cleft lip and pallet will need specialised feeding support from the beginning. Your hospital should be able to provide this for you, and there are charities available to support with general issues relating to clefts.

For the earliest babies, first feeds tend to be quite different to what you will probably have imagined. There will be lots of nudging, smelling, kneading, and licking from the baby before you can even consider 10-minute feeds. All these early experiences are invaluable, though. Each moment spent at or near a breast is a milestone in your journey all about learning how to feed and enjoy being close to you. Celebrate the small wins and know that time is on your side. For most premature babies, they will latch, given the time to grow and develop. Know that it is possible to mixed-feed long term, and do not be scared to stand up for your personal feeding goals. Sometimes staff wishes to have a neat box ticked, exclusive breastfeeding or formula-feeding. Know that you can, and many parents do, breastfeed for years while doing both.

If you are not feeling supported or getting the support you feel you should, you can ask to speak to the specialist breastfeeding professionals within your hospital. There might be an infant feeding coordinator, an IBCLC, or even a specialist feeding nurse/midwife within the unit. Many parents will also access phone/online support from other breastfeeding supporters who can give you both tips and validation while you are dealing with the emotional and physical demands of feeding your baby.

Emotional Health

During this stressful time, you may find some of the following helpful:

- ◊ Practice meditation or mindfulness.
- ◊ Find other parents with similar feeding goals.
- ◊ Rest when not with the baby.
- ◊ Get as much skin to skin as permitted.
- ◊ Participate in your baby's care.

How Much Milk

The medical and nursing team around your baby(s) will take the lead in working out volumes and often also a timetable for feeding times. It can often feel like you have little control over your baby's feeding, especially when they are sick or premature.

I encourage you to ask lots of questions. Ask to be involved and know this is your baby, and ultimately, you get the final say in what does and doesn't happen. You can usually offer time at the breast with every feed you are there for, although you might need to make it clear to the staff that this is your wish, and if there has been a shift change, you may well need to tell everyone you come across initially. Eventually, you will notice regular swallows and pauses in feeding. These pauses are normal and expected; babies need to take lots of breaks to breathe and rest, especially if they are small. The sucking bursts will get longer as the baby gets older and stronger.

The staff helping to care for your baby will calculate your baby's milk volumes based on their weight. Over the first few days, this increases until around day 3 when they need 150 ml/kg they weigh. This total is then divided up into the amount of feeds they have in 24 hours. Often, this will be a combination of your milk and either donor human milk or a formula.

Sometimes if babies need to catch up on growth, it might be recommended that they need more milk than 150 ml/kg, and you may also be offered something called a fortifier. Fortifier is added to human milk to provide extra fat. This does not mean that your milk is bad or not good enough. It just means that as well as your milk, your baby needs a little extra help.

Feeding your baby in the NICU can be confusing. But please know it will be a lot simpler to manage feeding at home with your baby. Once your baby is home, you may initially have some medication to add to the feeds, but soon, you will be feeding your baby just the same as other parents who are mixed-feeding.

You can see more about picking formulas on the First Steps Nutrition website, and the hospital staff will be able to guide you with the medical requirements. But the brand (if there is a choice) will be your choice alone.

Reducing top-ups will be guided by the hospital staff while the baby is under their care. When you are home with your baby, you will have more freedom regarding the pattern of the feeds, with many parents choosing to give some full breastfeeds and the bottled milk at only a few feeds a day. Even with a low milk supply, parents often say that this is easier than prepping bottles every feed.

Things to Be Aware of

◊ Giving formula while not expressing to maintain or build milk supply will only lead to less breastmilk being made.

◊ Seeking good support to help you with the underlying causes of low milk supply or slow weight gain is important if you want to return to exclusive breastfeeding. The Top Up Trap is not a fun place to be – you need to keep removing milk if you're giving top ups of formula or donated milk with a view to returning to full breastfeeding.

◊ Every single drop of human milk is incredibly helpful for your baby. This isn't an "all or nothing" situation.

Final Thoughts on Premature or Sick Babies

There is no doubt that feeding your baby through such challenging circumstances will be emotionally tiring as well as physically demanding. If you find yourself in a position where you are combination feeding, it is important to remember that this is beneficial, valid, and amazing. You are not failing your baby. If you want to work on increasing milk supply to provide more breastmilk, then please do read the info in Chapter 4, but if you've found a middle ground that protects your mental health, then that's fantastic, too.

Twins and Triplets (written by Kathryn Stagg, IBCLC)

There is little evidence regarding making enough milk for two or three babies. Milk supply works on a demand and supply basis. Having two or three babies coming to the breast means the breasts are stimulated two or three times more than those feeding a singleton. And so, they should produce two or three times the milk (Saint, 1986).

When I speak to expectant multiple parents, many assume that they will have to combination- feed. Our society, friends, family, and health professionals all believe it is difficult, even impossible, to make enough milk for more than one baby. However, with good breastfeeding support, and frequent and efficient feeds, most find they can make enough milk for their babies. I usually suggest giving breastfeeding a good go to start with, as it is far easier to move from breastfeeding to formula than from formula to breastfeeding.

Around 40% of twin babies, and nearly all triplets and higher-order multiples, are born prematurely or unwell and have to go to the neonatal unit. In this situation, the breastfeeding journey is started via expressing colostrum and breast milk and feeding via a tube. Frequent pumping with a hospital-grade double pump will give the best chance of establishing a copious supply (Hill et al., 2005). But as the babies grow and become more efficient feeders, milk supply is easier to establish. There seems to be little research into whether there is a window of opportunity to establish a full milk supply. It is certainly possible to increase milk volumes several months into their breastfeeding journey.

Most twins are born around 36 to 37 weeks gestation. This can mean they struggle initially as even though a twin pregnancy is deemed as "full term" at 37 weeks, the babies are not full-term babies. They can be quite small, sleepy, and inefficient on the breast to begin with (Ayton et al., 2012). These babies sometimes need topping up with expressed milk or formula after a feed to start off with, often called triple feeding. Parents start by breastfeeding the babies, topping up with expressed if they have it, or formula if they don't by the cup, syringe, or bottle, and then double pumping with a hospital-grade pump. They should be doing this eight times a day, every three hours. This is an intense regime and many struggle, especially with the pumping. As the babies approach 40-weeks gestation, they are often feeding more effectively, and top-ups can be gradually phased out.

Multiples that are born closer to full-term are likely to struggle less with breastfeeding. So, if the parents are supported to feed frequently with optimum positioning and attachment, the breasts should be stimulated sufficiently to make enough milk for more than one baby. Tandem feeding can often help make feeding more efficient and will help the parents cope with fussy behaviour and cluster feeding.

There may be a point where the family thinks they are at maximum capacity for breastfeeding and milk production, whether this is some time into the journey of establishing supply or after a full supply has been established. This can be because of physiological reasons of not being able to produce enough milk (this is actually pretty rare), a difficult start with breastfeeding where milk supply was never fully established, or for other reasons to do with mental overload. Combination-feeding can be a good option for these families. It is so important to value every drop of breast milk these families can give. Formula can be a good tool to prolong the breastfeeding relationship if used in a considered way.

So many families start by breastfeeding and then topping up with formula. However, this is not something that can be kept up long-term. Feeding both breast and bottle every feed can be too much work, especially once the partner has gone back to work. If there are physiological reasons for low supply, using a supplementary nursing system can be a great option. The babies can be topped up at the breast, and so the breastfeeding relationship is protected, and milk supply is maximised.

Many families prefer to give one or two set bottle feeds of formula a day and breastfeed responsively in between. This pattern is often suggested when the babies are struggling with weight gain, and some families choose to keep it long-term. It protects breastfeeding as long as the babies are being breastfed responsively the rest of the time, and the parents don't fall into "the top-up trap" when babies are fussy or feeding more frequently.

The top-up trap happens when babies need more milk, and more formula is offered, so babies come to the breast fewer times. This then means less milk is produced by the breast, which then means more formula is needed. And so on, until the babies begin to refuse the breast because of a low supply. Breastfeeding responsively in between the bottle-feeds prevents this from happening. If the bottle-feed can be given by someone other than the breastfeeding parent, this can be a good way of having a break, getting more sleep, or spending more time with older children.

For triplet families, and the twin-related scenarios discussed above, there is also the issue that there are more babies than breasts. Various patterns of breastfeeding, expressing, and formula-feeding can be adopted. Some triplet families prefer to breastfeed each baby individually. This becomes more doable as the babies become more efficient on the breast and feeds shorten. Many exclusively breastfeeding triplet families tandem feed two babies together, single feed the third, and rotate the pattern.

Some prefer to tandem feed two babies and feed the third expressed milk, pumping afterward for the next feed and rotating the pattern. Or they can single feed one baby and express for two. Some prefer to combination-feed with formula. They can tandem two babies and give formula to the third and rotate. They can single feed one baby and formula-feed the other two. Some prefer a similar pattern to twins where they exclusively breastfeed for some of the days and give a couple of set bottle-feeds. There are all sorts of combinations. And for higher-order multiples, similar patterns can be adopted.

Trauma and Your Breasts/Chest

Trauma around your breasts (or chest, if this is the language you use) is something we don't often discuss in our society. However, a history of sexual abuse or body dysmorphia (as is often experienced if you have an eating disorder, for example) are significant factors to have on your mind when considering how you might want to feed your baby. As discussed in the chapter on our society, these issues impact the trans community as well. For people falling into this category of holding some sort of trauma here, combination-feeding may prove to be a lifeline, as it can often feel more tolerable than exclusive breastfeeding.

Sometimes simply giving you back the power around your own body and what you choose to do with it can lift much of the fear and anxiety you may be experiencing. Combination- feeding might be as simple as "I breastfeed until it's too much… and then I give a bottle." It may be that instead, you need to know that you're going to breastfeed 4 times a day, or alternate between one bottle-feed and one breastfeed. There is no right or wrong here, and the choices you make will be deeply personal to you. I want you to know that this is okay.

If possible, it can be helpful to seek professional support from a therapist for the feelings that might come up while feeding your baby. Any of the techniques you already find helpful can be supportive here as well – mindfulness, distraction, or grounding exercises are all examples of this. But the possibilities are far greater. You may find that breastfeeding is an empowering, healing experience – but this isn't guaranteed. Neither is "right" or "wrong" These are simply your own unique experiences and a part of your life story. Get support. Know you are incredible. Be kind to yourself.

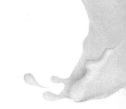

CHAPTER 11

Real Stories from Real Families

Giving voices to the families who have lived through combination-feeding is an important part of the discussion for me. In the following pages, you can find stories from several mothers who wanted to share their words here. They range from those who always wanted to combination-feed to those who needed to come to terms with mixed-feeding after wanting desperately to exclusively breastfeed. The words are all their own. I have only made grammatical and spelling changes.

Enjoy.

Louise's Story

I always knew I wanted to breastfeed my daughter. Having grown her for 9 months, developing a bond between us, and continuing to nurture her with my milk was something I was looking forward to. After a difficult birth, my milk took 5 days to come in, and breastfeeding wasn't as straightforward as I hoped.

My daughter lost over 10% of her birthweight, but I was repeatedly told that my latch "looked fine" and surely her birthweight would be regained soon. After 4 weeks of passing and her birthweight still not being reached, my daughter was admitted to hospital. The doctor told me, "It's time to be practical. You must give her formula." There was no further discussion about breastfeeding.

I felt like a total failure. I had tried so, so hard for the past month, but something just wasn't working. Had I been selfishly putting my desire to breastfeed above the healthy weight gain of my baby? Had I been starving her? After a traumatic birth, why had my body seemingly let my daughter down again? I was distraught. I have no family who breastfeeds, and while they meant well, their comments about "fed being best" really did not comfort me. It made me feel as if my grief about not successfully breastfeeding didn't matter.

The lack of understanding of why breastfeeding had not worked was tearing me apart. I sought out a local IBCLC with no expectation of being able to breastfeed again but to hopefully get some form of closure through understanding what had gone wrong. It turns out that my baby had a posterior tongue-tie, and I have insufficient glandular tissue in my breasts, probably connected to my polycystic ovaries. I always knew that my boobs looked a bit "different," but I had no expectation this would impact breastfeeding. Having this understanding as to why breastfeeding hadn't worked gave me comfort.

Following the release of my baby's tongue-tie, and with support from the IBCLC, we've been able to maximise the milk that I do have so that I can combination-feed my daughter. I see my feeding relationship with my daughter as predominantly breastfeeding her but providing her with some extra calories from formula to ensure she's getting all she needs. I was worried that my daughter would get a preference for bottles, but so far, she still looks to me for food and comfort. We're still going strong combination-feeding at 5 months, and I don't have any intention of stopping breastfeeding until my daughter wants to.

Madeline's Story

Our first son, Alex, was born in May 2017 by an emergency C-section. There was the first shock. My mum had given birth with (relative) ease to three children naturally, and so I wrongly assumed I'd do the same. But my baby had different ideas! I felt like a failure. When breastfeeding didn't work out (slow weight gain went un-investigated as I was in the throes of PND and didn't realise I could get help, so out came the formula), there were more feelings of failure. Of course, my mum had breastfed all three of us with no issues. Breastfeeding quickly petered out.

Our second son, Ted, was born in January this year with forceps, via the correct exit. Hurrah! Through EBF, he only lost 1% of his birthweight in the first week. Success! I was elated; everything was going well, and no sign of PND or anxiety. I was so proud of my body and mind.

Some weeks later, after mixed advice and opinions from several HVs and midwives following a reduced weight gain and incredibly regular feeding, we were finally referred to an IBCLC when Ted was 8 weeks old. She was incredible, quickly diagnosing posterior tongue-tie and a cows' milk protein allergy. We arranged for a private appointment to cut the tie (it was close to full lockdown, and we were unsure of whether we could have the procedure done through the NHS). All went well, and he seemed more settled.

Some weeks later, we suspected a second allergy and took him back to see the LC. His weight gain had dropped significantly as the tie had re-formed. We had slipped the HV net due to the lockdown, and so the weight gain drop had been missed. Our LC recommended significant top-ups with hypoallergenic formula immediately as it was becoming serious. I was heartbroken and felt huge guilt for not listening to my gut as he had still been feeding so often and had been awake every hour at night for weeks and weeks (I initially thought it was a bad case of the 4-month sleep regression).

As the next weeks passed and Ted visibly grew delightfully chubby and settled back into sleep(ish), I gradually learned to come to terms with combination-feeding as a long-term plan as it also seemed that I had low breast storage capacity. I learned not to see it as failure but progression and doing the best for our son after a run of bad luck. I stopped feeling like I was cheating for enjoying the advantages of combination-feeding.

I started enjoying breastfeeding again as it was no longer a 24/7 job and became pleasurable again. It hadn't been my choice or my fault, and we still enjoyed that closeness through breastfeeding, with Ted getting all those lovely booby benefits. No one could question our bond. With Ted now 20-weeks-old, whenever I have doubts, I think back to our LC commenting at one of our last appointments, "Just look at how much he loves you." The power of that observation will stay with me for a long, long time.

Rosie's Story

Dot was born a month early, but at 7 lbs 1 oz, she endured prematurity very well. However, she had little desire to feed. Other mums on the ward desperately soothed and fed endlessly. I had to strip Dot naked to wake her up enough to even look at my breast. It only took hours for her to feel floppy. The nurses pushed breastfeeding. But their methods of pinching my nipple and forcing it into Dot's mouth were of no help. Syringe feeding worked for a while, and cup feeding was okay, but after a couple of swallows, she would lose interest and dribble the milk out again. Clearly, she wanted to sleep for the extra month she had been promised.

But I wasn't worried. I was going to breastfeed. That was the plan.

The next day, her jaundice was worsening, and she would barely wake up. I was given the choice: tube feeding or a bottle.

I'm ashamed to say that bottles had been so criminalised in my mind that I considered tube feeding to protect our breastfeeding journey before I thought about Dot's own discomfort.

Dot took the bottle gladly, which was a good thing, but I remember feeling so inadequate, thoroughly unrequired.

Once home, I called Leigh, a breastfeeding consultant. I wasn't ready to give up breastfeeding, but I felt sure that I had ruined it.

But Leigh didn't deliver the guilt trip I was expecting. She taught us paced bottle-feeding, showed me a manageable pumping schedule, and set us off with a programme of breastwork.

Dot flourished with bottle-feeding. But I still felt guilty. How could I be feeding my baby this blank, faceless liquid when I had "gold" to give? I saw judgemental looks everywhere, assuming implied laziness instead of the true disappointment I felt. I hated buying formula.

Night after night of skin to skin, wrestling with an SNS, and an endless cycle of sterilising-pumping-feeding followed.

Then, at 1 month old, she just got it! I remember standing in the kitchen, and she wanted me. I gave her my breast, and she started feeding like a pro. We got straight into a cycle of actual breastfeeding, which, after a month of her barely putting my breast in her mouth at all, felt like a miracle.

We continued with regular bottles to manage her weight at first and then slipped into a natural cycle of combination-feeding, and it was great! Sharing the feeding gave me the freedom to sleep, to take a long shower, to go for a walk by myself while my husband could enjoy the unexpected daddy-daughter time that bottle-feeding gave him.

After a year, I was actually sad to pack up the bottles I had wept over months before. Looking back, I see that they were just a tool. They helped my baby when I couldn't, and they helped me to retain some independence when I needed it. Neither of us is any the worse for wear, and I wouldn't have changed a thing.

Conclusion

Thank you for picking up and reading this book. I sincerely hope that the words in these pages are helpful and reassuring. If you come away feeling supported, then *Mixed Up* has served its purpose. Every single parent I have ever met is doing their absolute best for their little ones, and it is always an honour to see the connection between parent and baby as they gaze into each other's eyes during a feed, regardless of whether that feed is from the breast or a bottle. All feeding deserves recognition and support. All parents are working hard.

Acknowledgements

A book like this is incredibly tricky to write. It is not a project I could have taken on alone. Of course, the first people who deserve to be acknowledged are the families who contributed both to the quotes and stories here and also who gave me the privilege of sharing time with them while they worked through their feeding challenges. I learn from every single dyad I meet or speak with, and this book exists because of each one of you.

Emma Pickett – Emma was the first person to see this book in its completed first draft state. Her way of offering constructive feedback was simply wonderful. Emma helped me to figure out the language and tone of this book as well as where some of the sections should go.

Dr Helen Crawley – Dr Crawley took the formula chapter and made it fit for use! Her expertise in the field of formula-feeding shines through in that part of the book, and I am incredibly grateful for her time and professionalism.

The contributors – Tessa, Kathryn, Anna, B. J., Leah, and Sarah – *thank you* for sharing your wisdom with me and those who pick up this book. I love that so much experience is weaved through the pages.

Lisa O'Sullivan– Lisa is single-handedly responsible for researching and writing up the individual ingredients in the breastmilk and formula. I paid her for this often-thankless work, but in hindsight, she might have preferred her long-dreamt-about woodchipper.

Victoria and Laine – For reminding me daily that I'm perfectly capable of doing all of the hard things. Also, for being The People in My Phone day and night.

Charlotte Bond – Charlotte has a talent for taking my atrocious grammar, rambling sentences, and love of "etc." and turning it all into a sensible piece of writing. She does so with humour and patience. Thank goodness for editors like Charlotte!

Alfie and Oliver - If it weren't for my experiences as a breastfeeding mum I wouldn't be an IBCLC today, and I certainly wouldn't be an author exploring infant feeding challenges! I hope as my boys grow up that they come to understand just how much they altered the path I was on for the better.

References

Aloe, L., Rocco, M. L., Balzamino, B. O., & Micera, A. (2015). Nerve growth factor: A focus on neuroscience and therapy. *Current Neuropharmacology, 13*(3), 294-303. doi:10.2174/1570159x13666150403231920

Association of Breastfeeding Mothers. (n.d.). *Team baby course.* Retrieved from: https://courses.abm.support/courses/team-baby-getting-ready-to-breastfeed/

Allers, K. S. (2017). *The big letdown: How medicine, big business, and feminism undermine breastfeeding* (1st ed.). St. Martin.

Ayton, J., Hanson, E., Quinn, S., & Nelson, M. (2012). Factors associated with initiation and exclusive breastfeeding at hospital discharge: late preterm compared to 37-week gestation mother and infant cohort. *International Breastfeeding Journal, 7*(16) Retrieved from https://internationalbreastfeedingjournal.biomedcentral.com/articles/10.1186/1746-4358-7-16

Biology.arizona.edu. (n.d.). *Amino Acids.* Retrieved from http://www.biology.arizona.edu/biochemistry/problem_sets/aa/aa.html

Bodnar, R. J. (2013). Epidermal growth factor and epidermal growth factor receptor: The yin and yang in the treatment of cutaneous wounds and cancer. *Advances in Wound Care (New Rochelle), 2*(1), 24-29. doi:10.1089/wound.2011.0326

Bonyata, K. (2018). Partial weaning and combination-feeding. Retrieved from https://kellymom.com/ages/weaning/wean-how/weaning-partial/

Boone, K. M., Geraghty, S. R., & Keim, S. A. (2016). Feeding at the breast and expressed milk feeding: Association with otitis media and diarrhea in infants. *Journal of Pediatrics, 174,* 118. doi:https://doi.org/10.1016/j.jpeds.2016.04.006) Vol 174 pages 118 - 125

Brown, A., & Harries, V. (2015). Infant sleep and night feeding patterns during later infancy: Association with breastfeeding frequency, daytime complementary food intake, and infant weight. *Breastfeeding Medicine, 10*(5), 246-252. https://doi.org/10.1089/bfm.2014.0153

Brown, A. (2019). *Why breastfeeding grief and trauma matter.* Pinter and Martin.

Centers for Disease Control and Prevention. (2018). *Public opinions about breastfeeding.* Retrieved from https://www.cdc.gov/breastfeeding/data/healthstyles_survey/index.htm

Cohen, M., & Otomo, Y. (2017). *Making milk.* Bloomsbury Publishing.

Davis, S.A, Knol, L.L., Crowe-White, K.M., Turner, L.W., & McKinley, E. (2020). *Homemade infant formula recipes may contain harmful ingredients: a quantitative content analysis of blogs.* Retrieved from https://pubmed.ncbi.nlm.nih.gov/32157977/

Da Silva Tanganhito, D., Bick, D., & Chang, Y. S. Breastfeeding experiences and perspectives among women with postnatal depression: A qualitative evidence synthesis. *Women Birth*, 33(3):231-239. doi: 10.1016/j. wombi.2019.05.012. Epub 2019 Jun 10. PMID: 31196830. Retrieved January 18, 2021 from https://pubmed.ncbi.nlm.nih.gov/31196830/

Dogaru, C. M., Nyffenegger, D., Pescatore, A. M., Spycher, B. D., & Kuehni, C.E. (2014). Breastfeeding and childhood asthma: Systematic review and meta-analysis. *American Journal of Epidemiology*, 179(10), 1153–1167, https://doi.org/10.1093/aje/kwu072

Drugs.com. (2020). *Moringa*. Retrieved from https://www.drugs.com/breastfeeding/moringa.html

Estrella, M. C., Mantaring J. B., David, G. Z., & Taup, M. A. (2000). A double-blind, randomized controlled trial on the use of malunggay (Moringa oleifera) for augmentation of the volume of breastmilk among non-nursing mothers of preterm infants. *Philippine Journal of Pediatrics, 49*, 3-6.

First Steps Nutrition Trust. (2020). *A simple guide to infant milks*. Retrieved from https://static1.squarespace.com/static/59f75004f09ca48694070f3b/t/5e81ea6e63d7965a88d492a0/1585572464338/Infant_milks_a_simple_guide_March2020.pdf

Fomon, S. (2001). Infant feeding in the 20th century: Formula and beikost. *Journal of Nutrition, 131*(2), 409S. doi: 10.1093/jn/131.2.409S. PMID: 11160571.

Garofalo, R. (2010). Cytokines in human milk. *Journal of Pediatrics, 156*(2 Suppl), S36-S40. doi: 10.1016/j.jpeds.2009.11.019. PMID: 20105664.

Geraghty, S. R., McNamara, K. A., Dillon, C. E., Hogan, J. S., Kwiek, J. J., & Keim, S. A. (2013). Buying human milk via the internet: Just a click away. *Breastfeeding Medicine, 8*(6), 474-478. doi: 10.1089/bfm.2013.0048.

Glasier, A., McNeilly, A. S., & Howie, P. W. (1984). The prolactin response to suckling. *Clinical Endocrinology, 21*, 109–116.

Greer, F. R., & Apple, R. D. (1991). Physicians, formula companies, and advertising. A historical perspective. *American Journal of Diseases of Childhood, 145*(3), 282-286. doi: 10.1001/archpedi.1991.02160030050019. PMID: 1781817.

Gulick, E. E. (1986). The effects of breast-feeding on toddler health. *Pediatric Nursing, 12*(1), 51-54. PMID: 3633073.

Haiden, N., Ziegler, E., & Ekhard, E. (2016). Human milk banking. *Annals of Nutrition and Metabolism, 69*(2), 8–15. doi:10.1159/000452821.

Hannan, A., Li, R., Benton-Davis, S., & Grummer-Strawn, L. (2005). Regional variation in public opinion about breastfeeding in the United States." *Journal of Human Lactation, 21*(3), 285-288

Hastrup. K. (1992). A question of reason: Breastfeeding patterns in seventeenth and eighteenth-century Iceland. *The Anthropology of Breastfeeding. Natural Law or Social Construct*, p. 91-108.

Health Development Agency. (2005). *UNICEF UK Baby Friendly Initiative, 2012*. Retrieved from https://www.unicef.org.uk/wp-content/uploads/sites/2/2013/09/baby_friendly_evidence_rationale.pdf

Hill, P. D., Aldag, J. C., Chatterton, R. T., & Zinaman, M. (2005). Primary and secondary mediators' influence on milk output in lactating mothers of preterm and term infants. *Journal of Human Lactation, 21*(2) 138-150.

Host, A., Husby, S., & Osterballe, O. (1988). A prospective study of cow's milk allergy in exclusively breast-fed infants: Incidence, pathogenetic role of early inadvertent exposure to cow's milk formula, and characterization of bovine milk protein in human milk. *Acta Paediatrica Scandanavica, 77*(5), 663-670.

Host, A., & Halken, S. (2014). Cow's milk allergy: Where have we come from and where are we going? *Endocr Metab Immune Disord Drug Targets, 14*(1), 2-8. doi: 10.2174/1871530314666140121142900.

Ip, S., Chung, M., Raman, G., Chew, P., Magula, N., DeVine, D., & Lau, J. (2007). *Breastfeeding and maternal and infant health outcomes in developed countries*. Evidence Report/Technology Assessment No.153AHRQ Publication No. 07-E007. Retrieved from http://www.ncbi.nlm.nih.gov/books/NBK38337/

Jewell, M., Edwards, C.M., Murphy, D. K., & Schumacher, A. (2019). Lactation outcomes in more than 3500 women following primary augmentation: 5-year data from the breast implant follow-up study. *Aesthetic Surgery Journal, 39*(8), 875-883. https://doi.org/10.1093/asj/sjy221

John, T. (2021). *Black mothers in the UK are four times more likely to die in childbirth than their White counterparts. Little is being done to find out why*. New York Times. Retrieved January 18, 2021 from https://www.cnn.com/2021/01/14/uk/uk-black-women-childbirth-intl-gbr/index.html

Kendall-Tackett, K., Cong, Z., & Hale, T. W. (2011). The effect of feeding method on sleep duration, maternal well-being, and postpartum depression. *Clinical Lactation, 2*(2), 22-26.

King, J., Raguindin, P. F., & Dans, L. (2014). *Moringa oleifera* (Malunggay) as a galactagogue for breastfeeding mothers: A systematic review and meta-analysis of randomized controlled trials. *The Philippine Journal of Pediatrics*. VL - 6 :323-4

Lane, H. (2020). *Medical bias, weathering and the deadly impact on Black mothers*. The Center for Community Solutions. Retrieved January 18, 2021 from https://www.communitysolutions.com/medical-bias-weathering-deadly-impact-black-mothers/

Lang, S., Lawrence C. J., & L'eorme. R. (1994). Cup feeding: An alternative method of infant feeding. *Archives of Diseases of Childhood, 71*(4), 365–369. doi: 10.1136/adc.71.4.365

Lauwers.J & Swisher.A Counselling the Nursing Mother (2015) Pg 521 Fig 22-29

Estrella, M. C., Bias, J., Taring, M. III, David, G.Z., & Taup, M.A. (2000). A double-blind, randomized controlled trial on the use of malunggay (Moringa oleifera) for augmentation of the volume of breastmilk among non-nursing mothers of preterm infants. *Philipp Journal of Pediatrics*, *49*, 3-6.

Mauch, C. E., Scott, J. A., & Magarey, A. M. (2012). Predictors of and reasons for pacifier use in first-time mothers: an observational study. *BMC Pediatrics*, *12*, 7. https://doi.org/10.1186/1471-2431-12-7

Mirkovic, K. R., Perrine, C. G., & Scanlon, K. S. (2016). Paid maternity leave and breastfeeding outcomes. *Birth: Issues in Perinatal Care*, https://doi.org/10.1111/birt.12230

Meier PP. Human Milk and Clinical Outcomes in Preterm Infants. Nestle Nutr Inst Workshop Ser. 2019;90:163-174. doi: 10.1159/000490304. Epub 2019 Mar 13. PMID: 30865984. Retrieved January 18, 2021 from https://pubmed.ncbi.nlm.nih.gov/30865984/

Mølbak, K., Gottschau, A., Aaby, P., Højlyng, N., Ingholt, L., & da Silva, A. P. (1994). Prolonged breastfeeding, diarrhoeal disease, and survival of children in Guinea-Bissau. *BMJ*, *308*(6941), 1403-1406. doi:10.1136/bmj.308.6941.1403

Monfu, M. (2020, February 4). I exclusively pumped—and there's not enough support for moms like me. Today's Parent Magazine. Retrieved January 18, 2021 from https://www.todaysparent.com/baby/breastfeeding/theres-not-enough-support-for-exclusive-pumping-moms/

Moro, G. E. (2018). History of milk banking: From origin to present time. *Breastfeeding Medicine*, *13*(S1), S16-S17.

Navarro-Rosenblatt, D., & Garmendia, M. (2018). Maternity leave and its impact on breastfeeding: A review of the literature. *Breastfeeding Medicine*, *13*(9), 589-597.

Neifert, M., DeMarzo, S., Seacat, J., Young, D., Leff, M., & Orleans, M. (1990). The influence of breast surgery, breast appearance, and pregnancy-induced breast changes on lactation sufficiency as measured by infant weight gain. *Birth*, *17*(1), 31-38. doi: 10.1111/j.1523-536x.1990.tb00007.x.

Noord C et al. Domperidone and ventricular arrhythmia or sudden cardiac death: a population-based case-control study in the Netherlands. Drug Saf. 2010 Nov 1; 33(11): 1003-1014.

Nowak, A.J., & Warren, J.J. (2000). Infant oral health and oral habits. *Pediatric Clinics of North America*, *47*(5), 1043-1066.

Onyango, A. W., Receveur, O., & Esrey, S. A. (2002). The contribution of breast milk to toddler diets in western Kenya. *Bulletin of the World Health Organization*, *80*(4), 292-299.

Owen, C., Whincup, P. H., Kaye, S. J., Martin, M. R., Smith Davey, G., Cook, D. G., et al. & Williams, S. M. (2008). Does initial breastfeeding lead to lower blood cholesterol in adult life? A quantitative review of the evidence. *American Journal of Clinical Nutrition*, *88*(2), 305-314. doi: 10.1093/ajcn/88.2.305.

Pearce, N., Ait-Khaled, N., Beasley, R., Mallol, J. K., Keil, U., Mitchell, E., & Robertson, C. (2007). "Worldwide trends in the prevalence of asthma symptoms: phase III of the International Study of Asthma and Allergies in Childhood (ISAAC)." *ISAAC Phase Three Study Group. Thorax, 62*(9), 758-766.

Perrin, M.T., Fogleman, A.D., Newburg, D.S., & Allen, J.C. (2017). A longitudinal study of human milk composition in the second year postpartum: implications for human milk banking. *Maternal/Child Nutrition, 13*(1), e12239. doi: 10.1111/mcn.12239.

Quigley, A., Kelly, Y., & Sacker, A. (2006). Breastfeeding and hospitalization for diarrheal and respiratory infection in the United Kingdom Millennium Cohort Study. *Pediatrics, 119*(4), e837-e842. DOI: https://doi.org/10.1542/peds.2006-2256

Radbill, S. X. (1981). Infant feeding through the ages. *Clinical Pediatrics, 20*(10), 613-621. doi:10.1177/000992288102001001

Radford, A (1991). *Breastmilk: A world resource*. Retrieved from: http://archive.babymilkaction.org/pdfs/worldresource91.pdf

Rossiter, M. D., Colapinto, C. K., Khan, M. K., McIsaac, J. L., Williams, P. L., Kirk, S. F., & Veugelers, P. J. (2015). Breast, formula and combination feeding in relation to childhood obesity in Nova Scotia, Canada. *Maternal/Child Health Journal, 19*(9), 2048-2056. doi: 10.1007/s10995-015-1717-y. PMID: 25656729.

Saint, L., Maggiore, P., & Hartmann, P.E. (1986). Yield and nutrient content of milk in eight women breastfeeding twins and one woman breastfeeding triplets. *British Journal of Nutrition, 56*(1), 49-58.

Scott KA, Britton L, McLemore MR. The Ethics of Perinatal Care for Black Women: Dismantling the Structural Racism in "Mother Blame" Narratives. J Perinat Neonatal Nurs. 2019 Apr/Jun;33(2):108-115. doi: 10.1097/JPN.0000000000000394. PMID: 31021935. Retrieved January 18, 2021 from https://pubmed.ncbi.nlm.nih.gov/31021935/

Sheehan, A., Gribble, K., & Schmied, V. (2019). It's okay to breastfeed in public but… *International Breastfeeding Journal, 14*(24). Retrieved from https://internationalbreastfeedingjournal.biomedcentral.com/articles/10.1186/s13006-019-0216-y

Simpson, E., Garbett, A., Comber, R. Madeline, B. (2016). Factors important for women who breastfeed in public: A content analysis of review data. *BMJ Open, 6,* e011762. doi: 10.1136/bmjopen-2016-011762

Speller, E., & Brodribb, W. (2012). Breastfeeding and thyroid disease: A literature review. *Breastfeeding Review, 20*(2), 41-47. PMID: 22946151.

Stevens, E. E. (2009). A history on infant feeding. *Journal of Perinatal Education, 18*(2), 32-39.

Stuebe, A. (2009). The risks of not breastfeeding for mothers and infants. *Reviews in Obstetrics and Gynecology, 2*(4), 222-231.

Tucker, C.M., Wilson, E. K., & Samandari, G. (2011). Infant feeding experiences among teen mothers in North Carolina: Findings from a mixed-methods study. *International Breastfeeding Journal, 6* (14). https://doi.org/10.1186/1746-4358-6-14

Turkyilmaz, C., Onal, E., Hirfanoglu, I. M., Turan, O., Koc, E., Ergenekon, E., & Atalay,Y. (2011). The effect of galactagogue herbal tea on breast milk production and short-term catch-up of birth weight in the first week of life. *Journal of Alternative & Complementary Medicine, 17*, 139-142.

van den Bogaard, C., van den Hoogen, H. J., Huygen, F. J., & van Weel, C. (1991). The relationship between breast-feeding and early childhood morbidity in a general population. *Family Medicine, 23*(7), 510-515. PMID: 1936731.

Vanky, E., Nordskar, J. J., Leithe, H., Hjorth-Hansen, A.K., Martinussen, M., & Carlsen, S. (2012). Breast size increment during pregnancy and breastfeeding in mothers with polycystic ovary syndrome: A follow-up study of a randomised controlled trial on metformin versus placebo. *BJOG: An International Journal of Obstetrics and Gynaecology.* doi: 10.1111/j.1471-0528.2012.03449.x

Vennemann, M.M., Bajanowski, T., Brinkmann, B., Jorch, G., Yücesan, K., Sauerland, C., &Mitchell, E.A. (2009). Does breastfeeding reduce the risk of sudden infant death syndrome? *Pediatrics, 123*(3), e406-410. doi: 10.1542/peds.2008-2145. PMID: 19254976.

Viggiano, D., Fasano, D., Monaco, G., & Strohmenger, L. (2004) Breastfeeding, bottle feeding, and non-nutritive sucking: Effects on occlusion in deciduous dentition. *Archives of Diseases of Childhood, 89*, 1121–1123. doi: 10.1136/adc.2003.029728

Wambach, K., & Riordan, J. (2016). *Breastfeeding and human lactation* (5th Ed). Jones & Bartlett Publishers.

Warren, J., Levy, S., Lester, K. H., Nowak, A., & Bergus, G. (2002). Pacifier use and the occurrence of otitis media in the first year of life. *Pediatric Dentistry, 103 - 107*

Weinberg, F. (1993). Infant feeding through the ages. *Canadian Family Physician, 39*, 2016-2020. PMID: 8219849.

White, N. (2020). *Revealed: The shocking healthcare racism endangering black mothers.* Huffington Post, UK. Retrieved January 18, 2021 from https://www.huffingtonpost.co.uk/entry/shocking-healthcare-racism-endangering-black-mothers_uk_5f2d3a2dc5b6b9cff7f0a3ba?guccounter=1

Wickes, I. G. (1953). A history of infant feeding. I. Primitive peoples; ancient works: Renaissance writers. *Archives of Diseases of Childhood, 28*(138), 151-158. doi: 10.1136/adc.28.138.151.

World Health Organization/UNICEF. (1989). Protecting, promoting and supporting breast-feeding. The *special role of maternity services: A joint WHO/UNICEF Statement.* Retrieved from https://www.who.int/nutrition/publications/infantfeeding/9241561300/en/

Wise, L. A., Titus-Ernstoff, L., Newcomb, P.A., Trentham-Dietz, A., Trichopouls, D., Hampton, J. H., & Egan, K. M. (2009). Exposure to breast milk in infancy and risk of breast cancer. *Cancer Causes and Control, 20*(7), 1083-1090.

Zimmerman, E., & Barlow, S. M. (2008). Pacifier stiffness alters the dynamics of the suck central pattern generator. *Journal of Neonatal Nursing, 14*(3), 79-86. doi:10.1016/j.jnn.2007.12.013

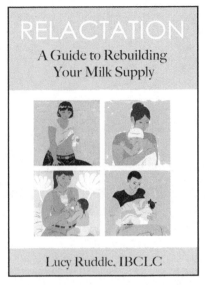

Made in the USA
Middletown, DE
21 April 2022

64592099R00119